Quality Reengineering in Health Care

Quality Reengineering in Health Care

The Clinical Laboratory of the University of Wisconsin Hospital and Clinics

RUSSELL TOMAR, MD
Professor, Pathology and Laboratory Medicine, Internal Medicine

JAMES WESTGARD, PhD
Professor, Pathology and Laboratory Medicine

ARTHUR EGGERT, PhD
Professor, Pathology and Laboratory Medicine

University of Wisconsin-Madison

ASCP
PRESS
American Society of Clinical Pathologists
Chicago

Publishing Team
Design and Production: Alan Makinen
Editorial: Ted Patla
Cover Design: Erik Tanck
Publisher: Joshua Weikersheimer

Library of Congress Cataloging-in-Publication Data
Tomar, Russell H.
    Quality reengineering in health care: the Clinical Laboratory of
    the University of Wisconsin Hospital and Clinics/Russell Tomar,
    James Westgard, Arthur Eggert.
            p.   cm.
    Includes bibliographical references.
    ISBN 0-89189-435-7 (alk. paper)
    1. Hospitals--Administration. 2. Total quality management.
3. Hospital laboratories--Administration. I. Westgard, James O.,
1941–   . II. Eggert, Arthur A., 1944–   . III. Title.
    [DNLM: 1. University of Wisconsin Hospital & Clinics. Clinical
Laboratory. 2. Total Quality Management--methods. 3. Laboratories,
Hospital--organization & administration--United States. 4. Models,
Organizational. 5. Organizational Innovation. WX 207 T655q 1998]
RA972.T65 1998
362.1'1'068—dc21
DNLM/DLC
for Library of Congress   98-7848
                                                                    CIP

03 02 01 00 99   5 4 3 2 1

Contents

Chapter 6.
LESSONS LEARNED *151*

Appendix *159*

Strategic Planning

INTRODUCTION

As a nation, we spend about 14% of our gross national product on health care, which makes the United States the world leader in health care expenditures. Furthermore, as we care for an aging population, expenses will continue to rise as newer and increasingly expensive medical technologies become available. The only checks to these rising costs involve rationing care and gaining efficiency.

For more than 10 years, clinical laboratories have had to deal with restrictions in reimbursement. The first blow at their economic viability occurred when changes in reimbursements were included in the Deficit Reduction Act (DEFRA) of 1984 and continued with the Consolidated Omnibus Budget Reconciliation Act (COBRA) of 1986 and the Omnibus Budget Reconciliation Acts (OBRAs) of 1987, 1989, 1990, and 1993. Laboratories were already faced with decreasing payments when the federal statute called the Clinical Laboratory Improvement Act of 1988 (CLIA-88) was enacted. CLIA places all clinical laboratories under federal regulation and requires federal inspection and accreditation.[1] By 1988, laboratorians were well aware of an imminent financial crunch since payments were being reduced as administrative costs were rising to meet the myriad of federal regulations.

Laboratorians were well aware of an imminent financial crunch since payments were being reduced as administrative costs were rising.

During this period, the need for increased productivity was not confined to the health care industry. The nation's industrial base had been declining for perhaps 25 years, and Japan, once mocked for its inferior workmanship, was not only making products cheaper, but also making them better, more reliable, and easier to use. As analysts in the United States examined the Japanese "miracle," they were shocked to learn that an American industrial statistician, J. Edwards Deming, was considered to be the Moses who led the Japanese into the new promised land of industrial superiority. Moreover, it was discovered that Deming's teachings had been rejected in this country more than 30 years earlier! Deming's philosophy of management,[2,3] called total quality management (TQM), is an extension of his early work into the quality control of manufacturing processes. TQM has since been adopted by many of the largest US companies and is a major reason for America's current economic resurgence.

The automotive industry is just one dramatic example of an industry adopting Deming's ideas. Conversely, the Joint Commission on Accreditation of Hospitals (JCAH), with its emphasis on "appropriateness" or utilization, outcomes, and inspection rather than process and customer satisfaction, was out-of-step until 1985 when the health care industry began to accept the tenets of TQM—carefully determining customer requirements, providing products and services that conform to those requirements, and improving productivity by eliminating problems in production processes. Our experience at the clinical laboratory of the University of Wisconsin Hospital and Clinics (UWHC) is an example of TQM as applied in the health care and public service sectors.

Our clinical laboratory began to explore the concepts and philosophy of TQM in the mid 1980s and began to implement it formally in the late 1980s. By that time, although JCAH had adopted the principles of TQM, we suffered several setbacks in our early efforts because of JCAH accreditation guidelines.

Meantime, customers were making increasing demands on clinical laboratories in terms of volume, variety, and quality of testing. Generally, clinical laboratories kept up with demand by automating as many of their procedures as quickly as possible. In so doing, laboratories were able to restrain the growth of costs. Furthermore, because laboratorians are experienced in dealing with new technology, clinical laboratories were among the first health care units to capitalize on the power of computers, initially as an electronic record but later as a monitor of quality control efforts.

Reengineering advocates examining and changing a whole system or process.

Over the last few years, the health care industry has turned to "reengineering" as another approach to improve its productivity and gain a competitive edge in the global marketplace. While TQM focuses on discrete improvements in an existing system, often initiated at any level in an organization, "reengineering," as described by Hammer and Champy,[4] advocates examining and changing a whole system or process. It proposes radical redesign of business processes for dramatic improvement. We initiated a reengineering program after the processes and values of TQM were well accepted in our clinical laboratory.

These pioneering efforts, however, should not be limited only to clinical laboratories but should be applied to the health care sector in general. These efforts were successful at improving and changing the clinical laboratory of the UWHC and will provide a practical guide for other laboratories that are considering or are initiating programs of change. We will describe our approaches, present our materials, and analyze our approaches, including revealing the lessons we have learned from our experiences.

BACKGROUND

Laboratory automation and computing have historically been areas of strength for the clinical laboratory at the UWHC. The importance of these areas was recognized in the 1960s, and a staff of analytical bio-chemists was assembled from recent graduates of doctoral programs on the Madison campus. They were involved in the early development and testing of automated systems and laboratory information systems. The Dupont aca™ (Dupont, Wilmington, Del) had close ties to the UWHC from its initial concept through the development of the chemical meth-ods and the testing of prototypes and production models. The LCI Labcom™ (LCI, Madison, Wis) laboratory information system evolved from prototypes that were developed and implemented at the university. Because of this background and these interests, the laboratory has often been involved in the testing, evaluation, and implementation of new laboratory systems.

The UWHC Clinical Laboratory had been formed as a hospital department rather than an academic unit. Because the director who led the laboratory during much of its early history was an internist, most of the laboratory faculty was part of internal medicine. In the late 1970s, most of the laboratory faculty moved to the department of pathology of the medical school; however, several of the laboratory faculty members, including the director, retained their tenure homes in other depart-ments, particularly internal medicine, and were granted joint or affiliate appointments in pathology.

The UWHC Clinical Laboratory had been formed as a hospital department rather than an academic unit.

The laboratory was segmented into sections or what the hospital called "cost centers." Chemistry, microbiology, hematology, blood bank, special chemistry, data processing, quality control, immunology, adminis-tration, and histocompatibility were individual cost centers. The hema-tology and blood bank section directors were MDs; however, the other sections were usually directed by PhDs.

The laboratory director met with each of the section directors every other week. Common meetings for all sections were rare. Decisions were made by the director or the associate medical director, who was also director of hematology. The director reported to a hospital associate superintendent or the superintendent directly. There were no regularly scheduled meetings between the laboratory and hospital administration.

Although most sections of the laboratory were physically adjacent in about 28,000 square feet on the second floor of the hospital, there were, for historical or pragmatic reasons, sections scattered throughout the building. The outpatient phlebotomy station and laboratory were in another module on the second floor; the blood bank was next to the operating rooms on the third floor; diagnostic immunology was on the fourth floor; trace metal analysis was on the fifth floor; gynecological endocrinology was on the sixth floor; and histocompatibility was about to be moved to the seventh floor. The total allotted space was adequate for the assigned activities.

The 1988–1989 budget included 191.58 full-time employees with total costs including personnel and supplies of $13,728,474 and revenue after deductions of $23,676,760. The annual capital equipment budget varied between $400,000 and $600,000. The laboratory performed 4,779,572 tests annually. During the late 1980s, the clinical laboratory at the UWHC comprised many different laboratories, each a minor fiefdom with its own management structure, budget, personnel, quality standards, and modes of operation.

The initial impetus behind the adoption of TQM was begun in 1985, when the JCAH began to push hospitals to establish a more structured and formal quality assurance program. Its accreditation manual introduced a new standard for pathology and laboratory medicine, requiring that, as part of the hospital's quality assurance program, the quality and appropriateness of pathology and medical laboratory services be monitored and evaluated and identified problems be resolved. These changes forced our clinical laboratory to examine and evaluate its quality program and explore directions for future development.

Following Juran's teachings,[5-7] we began a series of pilot projects to learn quality improvement methodology; to determine whether it would work in a health care facility; to demonstrate management commitment to quality improvement; and to provide a broader, laboratory-wide orientation and perspective for our section-oriented faculty, directors, managers, and supervisors.

J. M. Juran, PhD, has been one of the leaders in quality management since the early 1950s, when he started working with the Japanese industry to develop approaches for participative management. Dr Juran is given much of the credit for setting the stage for the development of quality circles in Japan and for developing the process and methodology for quality improvement project teams in the United States. He is a prolific writer and also the founder of The Juran Institute, which provides training courses, training materials, and consultation services to hundreds of companies and organizations.

As stated earlier, in the mid 1980s, the only documented examples of TQM were coming from industry, and the general attitude in health care was that "we are different" and industrial approaches for quality improvement did not apply to us. It was not yet readily apparent to health care providers that the examples discussed by industry actually represented the same kinds of problems we faced in health care. However, it was easier for laboratories to see that production-oriented industrial approaches should be applied to the production of test results[8]; after all, we had already adopt-

The clinical laboratory at the UWHC comprised many different laboratories, each a minor fiefdom with its own management structure.

The general attitude in health care was that "we are different."

ed statistical process control approaches that were originally developed in industry. Nevertheless, there still was a lot of skepticism that needed to be overcome by proving that the principles, concepts, and methodology of industrial quality improvement would work in the laboratory.

CHARGE TO THE NEW DIRECTOR

On the laboratory director's pending retirement in 1988, the chair of pathology, the hospital superintendent, and the dean of the medical center formed a medical-center–wide search committee that recruited the laboratory's next laboratory director, who reported to the chair and the superintendent. He was given the following ground rules: all academic appointments, promotions, and raises went through the department and the chair while budgets and daily operations went through the hospital superintendent. All funds generated by the laboratory went to the hospital or the department. There were no flexible funds available to the laboratory or its director.

The new director was charged with developing a more professional service organization and increasing its academic productivity. Hospital administration expected the laboratory to improve or maintain service, ie, turnaround times and menu selection; become more customer-focused; and improve its productivity, ie, cost-effectiveness. The department expected the laboratory to provide a milieu whereby academic output would increase.

The new director was charged with developing a more professional service organization and increasing its academic productivity.

TOTAL QUALITY MANAGEMENT BACKGROUND

Madison is and has been a center for TQM. The mayor of Madison in the 1980s, Joe Sensenbrenner, had embraced it. Several state agencies were advocating its use. The chancellor of the University of Wisconsin-Madison, Donna Shalala, had hired a lobbyist whose background was in the city's TQM programs. The quality control section of the laboratory had piloted educational efforts in this type of management. Thus, we were aware of the principles of TQM, which appeared to us as the scientific method applied to management.

The clinical laboratory's pilot projects in 1985 included development of a computer program to monitor the turnaround times of laboratory tests[9], the design of quality control procedures to optimize the quality and productivity of high-volume multitest chemistry analyzer[10], introduction of a newsletter to communicate changes in laboratory services to our users, and development of a standard policy and procedure for correcting test reports. This variety of projects allowed us to study different types of processes from technical to nontechnical, establish within-section and across-section laboratory project teams, and consider the quality requirements of both internal and external customers.

The principles of TQM appeared to us as the scientific method applied to management.

From these early experiences as well as our study of the available TQM literature, we began to formalize a problem-solving model that included six steps. First, problem selection needed to consider the customers affected, time required, resources required, and the needs and capabilities of the team. Second, the need for a short-term or quick fix had to be assessed before development of a long-term solution. Third, the root cause of the problem had to be determined. Fourth, a solution had to be identified. Fifth, a solution had to be implemented and documented. Sixth, the implemented solution had to be evaluated to be sure it solved the original problem.

To support the team, we had one person trained as a quality-circle facilitator who was able to identify the tools and techniques that would be appropriate and who would help the pilot teams with their applications. We employed common group-oriented problem-solving tools and techniques, such as brainstorming, nominal group, flowcharting, Pareto diagrams, cause and effect or fishbone (also called "Ishikara" after the developer of this tool) diagrams, and force-field analysis.

A Framework for Quality Management

The scientific method is basic to the TQM approach, which is often described by the following steps: Plan a study, Do the experiment, Check the data to see what happened, then Act on that data (PDCA). This PDCA cycle is often repeated as new information leads to new questions that must be answered by another experiment before a problem can be finally solved. Because most laboratorians are trained as scientists, it seemed natural and logical to adopt a scientific method as our quality management model.[11-13] We recast the PDCA cycle as the quality management framework shown in Figure 1-1, where the components represent quality planning (QP), quality laboratory processes (QLP), quality control (QC), quality assessment (QA), and quality improvement (QI). Central to this quality management framework are the goals, objectives, and quality requirements to be achieved by the laboratory.

In this 5-Q framework, QLP represents the policies, procedures, practices, and people that establish the processes that get the work done. QC represents direct measures of process performance with short feedback times that allow the laboratory to evaluate whether certain aspects of quality are satisfactory, particularly analytical quality as monitored by statistical quality control. QA represents quality assessment by other measures, usually with longer feedback times and loops that allow the laboratory to measure quality only after the service has been delivered—turnaround time of a test, for example. QI means quality improvement, and in a broad sense, includes improvements made by individuals and by project teams. In most laboratories, the biggest need

We recast the PDCA cycle as the quality management framework.

Central to the quality management framework are the goals, objectives, and quality requirements to be achieved by the laboratory.

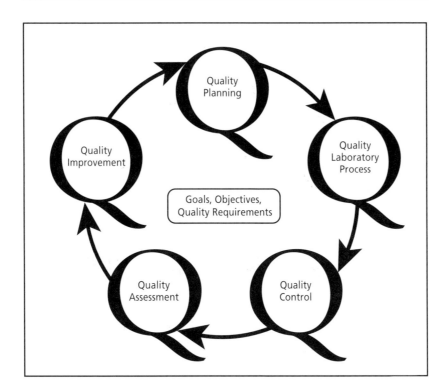

Figure 1-1.
5-Q framework for managing quality.

is to provide an effective team problem-solving mechanism to tackle those problems that cross organizational boundaries. QP stands for quality planning, which should be the starting point for managing and implementing quality laboratory processes, but Juran indicates that planning is usually learned by improving processes and making changes to existing processes by re-planning.

This 5-Q framework provides a management process that can be applied by individuals in their own work, by teams in project work, and by management itself. Individuals usually own, that is, control, small subprocesses in which they can identify problems and make improvements, whereas the ownership of larger processes usually involves many individuals and often more than one department, thus requiring a team approach. Large improvements, such as those targeted by reengineering, require management itself to lead the planning effort. This 5-Q framework also helps people understand how the apparent conflict between standardized work processes and continual improvements in those processes can coexist.

Quality assurance is the outcome of this whole process, rather than being a component for measuring quality, which is identified as quality assessment in the 5-Q framework. Measuring some characteristics of quality does not in any way guarantee that the necessary quality has or

This 5-Q framework provides a management process that can be applied by individuals in their own work, by teams in project work, and by management itself.

Quality assurance is the outcome of this whole process.

will be achieved, any more than measuring productivity somehow improves productivity; however, it is required before one can systematically tackle quality improvement.

Piloting Quality Improvement Projects

In assessing the weaknesses of traditional laboratory quality management practices based on the 5-Q framework, three needs stood out as having high priority—quality improvement, quality planning, and quality goals. Given Juran's advice that quality planning is best learned through quality improvement and the replanning of processes, we adopted as our basic strategy Juran's project-by-project improvement approach[6] for developing the quality improvement component of our quality management process.

Quality planning is best learned through quality improvement and the replanning of processes.

Quality improvement, in this context, emphasizes problem solving by a team of process owners (the people involved in the work). Processes are imperfect and need to be improved to eliminate problems and prevent recurrences, which will improve quality. Every repeated activity in the laboratory is a process; therefore, virtually all laboratory problems are process problems and subject to the same quality improvement methodology. What differs from problem to problem is the nature of the process (the work to be accomplished) and its ownership. According to Juran, chronic problems often exist because no single person is responsible for that work and, therefore, no single person is able to solve that problem. What is needed is a team-oriented approach that involves all the individuals who have ownership of the process. The key techniques we employed are described below.

- *Brainstorming* is an interactive group technique for generating a list of ideas in response to a stated question or problem. Ideas are collected from team members in rotation, one idea per turn, until everyone has finished contributing. The ideas are then discussed and prioritized by voting.

- *Nominal group* is similar to brainstorming, but the question is posed in advance to allow some time for individuals to generate a list of ideas. These ideas can be collected at a team meeting or via mail, telephone, or e-mail, though these latter collections lose the spontaneity and creativity that may occur when done at a team meeting. The ideas or items are then discussed and prioritized by voting.

- *Flowcharting* means drawing a diagram that maps the sequence and relationships of steps in a process.

- *Pareto diagram* refers to a histogram with intervals rearranged to show groups in order from highest to lowest frequency of observations, often frequency of problems.

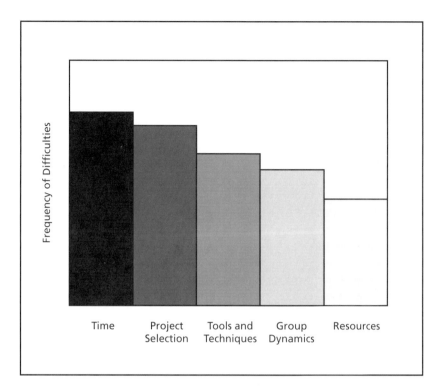

Figure 1-2.
Pareto diagram show-ing difficulties experi-enced with pilot projects (from *Lab Med.* 1989;20:243, with permission).

- *Cause-and-effect diagram* is also commonly known as a *fish-bone diagram* because it converts a list of items to a graphic display that looks like the skeleton or bones of a fish. This is often used to organize a list of possible causes under headings such as materials, methods, machines, and manpower.

- *Force-field analysis* is a technique for identifying both the positive and negative factors (driving and restraining forces) that affect the level of performance or the achievement of a goal.

Our experiences with these pilot projects from 1985 through 1988 were both productive and frustrating. Although each project had a successful conclusion, we identified a number of difficulties, as shown by the Pareto diagram in Figure 1-2. We found that the time required for project-by-project improvement was much greater than we anticipated, careful guidance on project selection was critical for timely resolution of problems, training was needed in the tools and techniques of TQM if the group was to work effectively, group dynamics were often critical for the success of the project, and resources had to be committed to the quality improvement projects if they were to succeed.

Selection of a "doable" project was much more difficult than we expected.

Selection of a "doable" project was much more difficult than we expected. Many factors needed to be considered, with particular attention being paid to customer focus, time for completion, resources needed, and team needs, as shown by the fishbone diagram in Figure 1–3. A narrow mission was important for new and inexperienced teams. Difficult projects required more seasoned team members who already understood the team process and had the skills and ability to work effectively in a group. The team charged with finding a method of recording continuing education for the laboratory staff had a well-defined, narrow mission and achieved its mission relatively quickly. The team charged with improving external communications spent considerable time in understanding the extent of its charge.

Full-scale implementation required a careful plan with stages or phases of activities.

Full-scale implementation required a careful plan with stages or phases of activities, as shown by the flowchart in Figure 1–4. Initial management activities required development of a formal quality policy, mission and values statements, a quality plan, pilot projects for success stories, a quality training program, and a recognition program. In the second phase, project teams were established to tackle management's agenda of problems. We anticipated that voluntary teams, like quality circles, would develop later and would work more directly on the agenda of the workers themselves. Finally, a mechanism for involvement of individuals directly in quality improvement was needed, which could employ a suggestion program, as well as what later developed to be "daily management."

A major management decision was made on whether to implement the new quality management process. An assessment of the forces at the time is shown by the force-field diagram in Figure 1–5. This force field analysis is almost 10 years old now, but still reflects many of the same forces present in the current health care and laboratory environment.

Today there is an even greater need for process improvements through TQM and major system changes through reengineering.

Today there is an even greater need for process improvements through TQM and major system changes through reengineering because the cost pressure is higher.

LONG-RANGE PLANNING

One of the difficulties in implementing TQM is getting upper management interested and involved in team-oriented activities that are important in their own work. The need to develop a long-range strategic plan for the laboratory provided us an opportunity to use a team process and many of the quality improvement tools in a project that was critical for its future direction and management. We seized this opportunity to apply the quality improvement methodology to develop a strategic plan.[14]

Apply the quality improvement methodology to develop a strategic plan.

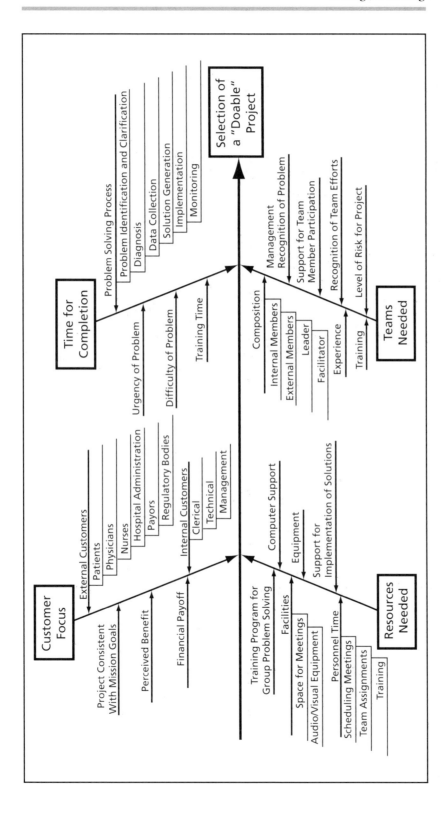

Figure 1-3.
Fishbone diagram showing factors to consider in selecting a "doable" project (from *Lab Med.* 1989;20:242, with permission).

Figure 1-4.
Flowchart showing plan for implementing a quality improvement program (from *Lab Med.* 1989;20:244, with permission).

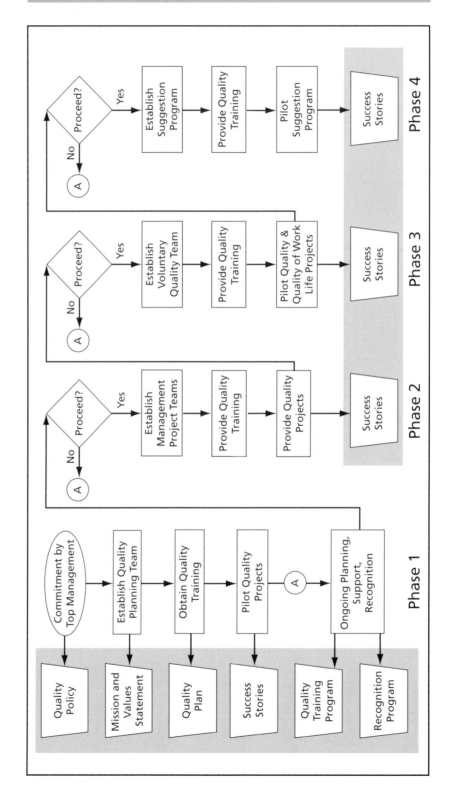

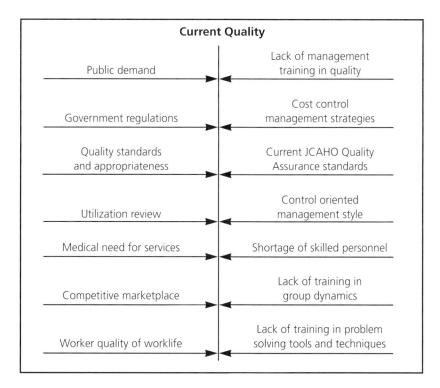

Figure 1-5.
Force-field analysis
showing driving and
restraining forces for
implementing a quality
improvement program
(from *Lab Med.* 1989;20:
246, with permission).

Current Quality

Public demand	Lack of management training in quality
Government regulations	Cost control management strategies
Quality standards and appropriateness	Current JCAHO Quality Assurance standards
Utilization review	Control oriented management style
Medical need for services	Shortage of skilled personnel
Competitive marketplace	Lack of training in group dynamics
Worker quality of worklife	Lack of training in problem solving tools and techniques

Objectives

We sought to improve the service of the clinical laboratory, making it more customer-focused and cost-effective, and increase its academic output to a position of leadership among other clinical laboratories.

The Long-Range Planning Team

The new laboratory director held meetings with each member of the management staff. There seemed to be little understanding or agreement as to the future direction of the clinical laboratory. From these discussions, the laboratory director became convinced that the laboratory and hospital needed a plan and that we should begin the process through a *long-range planning team*.

The decision to form such a team was an easy one; however, determining its composition proved a more difficult proposition. Conventional wisdom suggested that the team should have no more than six to eight members, but we felt that all or almost all elements should be represented. Because the laboratory was splintered into more than a dozen independent units, it was recognized that these units were somewhat competitive with each other, and many of them would be uncomfortable being represented by someone from another center. It was deter-

There had to be "buy-in" to the new program.

mined that the team would have to be expanded to include almost all sections for input and "buy-in" to the new program. We believed that the faculty/section directors as well as the medical technologists needed to be represented. We also sought individuals who had demonstrated the capacity to work well in a group. In addition, we asked hospital administration and the chair of pathology for representatives.

After considerable debate, the team was named and consisted of six section directors including the director of the clinical laboratory, five technologists, and one hospital administrator. The director of quality assurance served as chair, while a medical technologist, the manager of the quality assurance section who was also a trained TQM facilitator, served as recording secretary. There was also clerical support to provide for the rapid writing and distribution of minutes and other materials. In addition, the chair and secretary also acted as facilitators by providing technical support in using group problem-solving tools and techniques and by identifying problems in group dynamics. Most of the sections had direct representation.

The Planning Process

The long-range planning team met 10 times between October 3 and December 20, 1988. Each meeting was scheduled for 1 to 2 hours. At the first meeting, ground rules were established (Table 1-1) and the planning/improvement process was described. We adopted a planning process from Holmberg (steps 1-5)[15] and Folger (step 6)[16] and a combination of the two for steps 7 and 8 (Figure 1-6). We brainstormed to collect ideas and then developed fishbone diagrams to make pictorial summaries of the results. At or before each meeting, reading materials were distributed to illustrate the specific tasks or processes under discussion. Thus, the long-range planning team became the first laboratory group to be instructed in the philosophy and methodologies of TQM. This was an important step because the team members were also the leaders of the laboratory.

The long-range planning team became the first laboratory group to be instructed in the philosophy and methodologies of TQM.

During our second meeting, we developed a list of laboratory customers, prioritized them, and identified their needs. We questioned if these needs were changing and if so, what new requirements must be considered for the future. This was put into fishbone format (Figure 1-7).

We followed this pattern in the next two meetings by brainstorming (1) future issues and trends that would affect the laboratory and (2) strengths/weaknesses and opportunities/threats, then placing them in fishbone diagrams (Figures 1-8 and 1-9).

After the first fishbone diagram, team members volunteered to work with the recording secretary to prepare the fishbone summary for

GROUND RULES FOR MEETINGS

Table 1-1.

1. The meetings will begin at the scheduled time.

2. Team members will attend all meetings unless out of town or ill.

3. Members will take measures to avoid pages or phone calls during meetings.

4. A quorum of eight members must be present for a meeting to take place.

5. Consensus positions will be established by a two-thirds vote of the members, with a minimum of six votes being necessary. A minority position can be stated when there is strong disagreement.

6. A participative process will be used; brainstorming will be a primary tool. Members are to be reminded of the rules of brainstorming, particularly the important step of collecting ideas without discussion or criticism.

7. Discussions of the committee will be considered open unless a specific item or topic is identified as confidential.

8. Minutes will be provided by someone external to the committee, rather than by assignment to a member of the committee.

9. Articles and materials will be circulated to the committee as part of the committee work. The team chair asks that any materials be given to him so that he can ensure that the laboratory director has a chance to preview the materials before distribution.

10. Agendas will be provided before each meeting.

11. Meetings will end at the scheduled time, unless there is a consensus agreement to extend the meeting because of the discussion in progress.

---

the next session. This provided another opportunity for training team members in TQM techniques.

The long-range planning teams had diagrams describing customers and their perceived needs, listing future issues and trends, and analyzing strengths/weaknesses and opportunities/threats (SWOT). It was not possible to engage all issues raised by these exercises. Thus, we sharpened our focus by assigning two to three members of the long-range planning teams to one of three subgroups to prioritize the materials in each of the three diagrams. These documents were then brought back to the whole committee for further discussion and eventual scoring by a nominal voting technique whereby all members graded each item and priorities were established by the sums. All three groups listed *ambulatory, reference,* and *off-site testing* as future areas that would have major impact on the laboratory. The following were named by two different groups: *cost containment, personnel shortages, quality and timeliness of reports,* and *research* that we would need to address as areas. *Changes in technology, space, interdepartment communication,* and *education* were each named by a single group. In this way, we were able to focus our initial efforts on some aspects of these nine issues.

Developing the Mission Statement

The planning team was now ready to develop a mission statement. The chair provided background materials including mission statements from our parent institution, the University of Wisconsin; our hospital organization, the UWHC; a neighboring hospital; and a few examples from industry. Morrisey's[17] reason for a mission statement gave us direction: ". . . an organization's mission statement describes the nature and concept of the organization's future business. It establishes what the organization plans to do and for whom, plus the major philosophical premises under which it will operate. This statement forms the foundation for the rest of the strategic and operational plans and provides a common vision for the total organization. . . ."

An organization's mission statement describes the nature and concept of the organization's future business.

To focus the team further, we asked team members to answer the following questions:

- Why do you work here rather than another laboratory?

- What makes you proud to be part of our laboratory?

- What should our laboratory stand for, be known for?

After collecting these thoughts, the team discussed the format of the mission statement. Then, all were asked to compose 5-minute drafts for the three mission subparagraphs of service, research, and education. These were presented to the whole group, clarified, and discussed. The laboratory director and the director of quality assurance were charged with drafting a mission statement consistent with those of our parent organizations and incorporating the ideas raised in the team discussion.

The draft was presented at the next meeting. Over the next 4 to 5 weeks, team members as well as many other laboratory and hospital employees provided insights and comments on the statement. A statement was approved by the team to be presented to the rest of the laboratory faculty, managers, and supervisors. A final version was adopted in December 1988 (Figure 1-10).

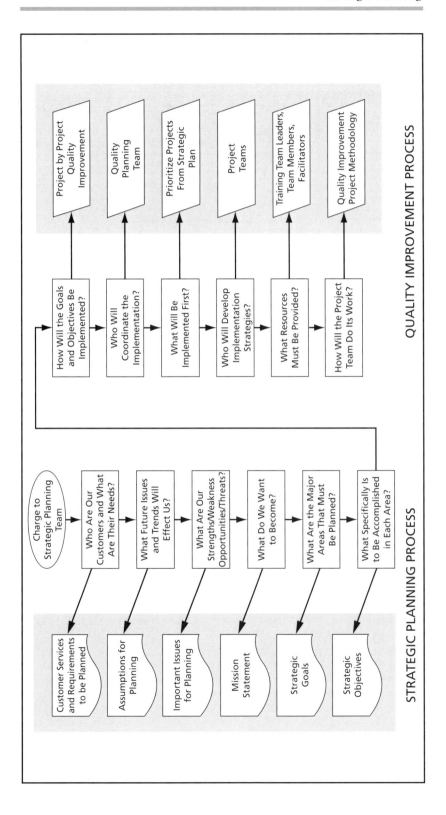

Figure 1-6.
Flow diagram of the planning process (from *CLMR*. 1991;5:363, with permission).

Figure 1.7
Fishbone diagram summarizing customers and their needs (from *CMLR*. 1991;5:364, with permission). JCAHO: Joint Commission on Accreditation of Healthcare Organizations; MT = medical technology; HMO = Healthcare maintenance organizations; CAP = College of American Pathologists; CLIA = Clinical Laboratory Improvement Act; HCFA = Health Care Financing Administration; QA = quality assessment; LID = laboratory information document; OP = outpatient

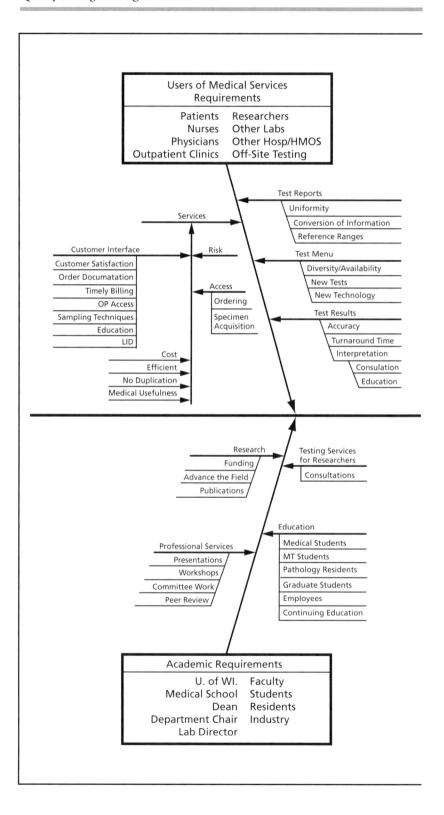

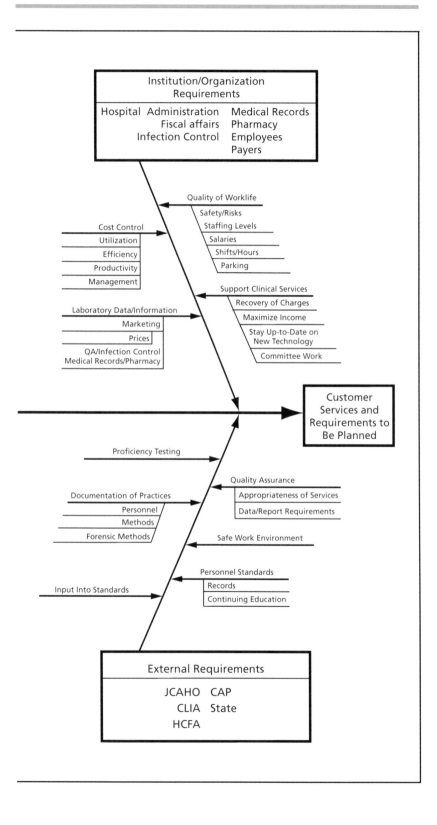

Figure 1.8.
Fishbone diagram summarizing future issues and trends (from *CLMR.* 1991;5:365, with permission). QC = quality control

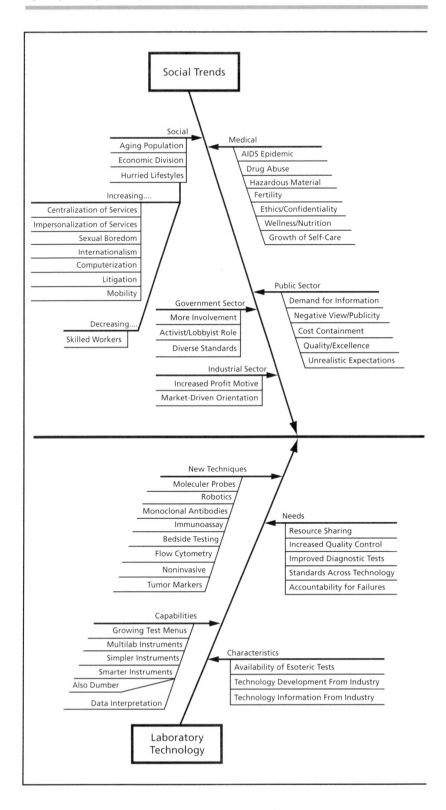

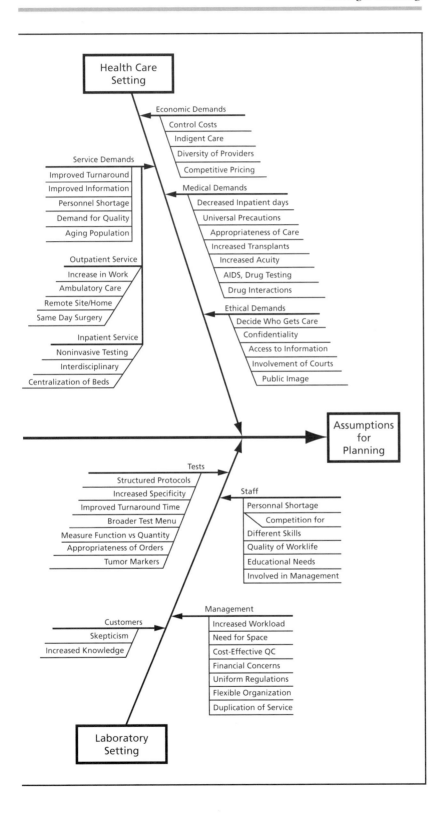

Figure 1-9.
Fishbone diagram summarizing SWOT analysis (from *CLMR* 1991a; 5:366, with permission). DRG = diagnostic related groups; Lab Med = laboratory medicine; OP = outpatient.

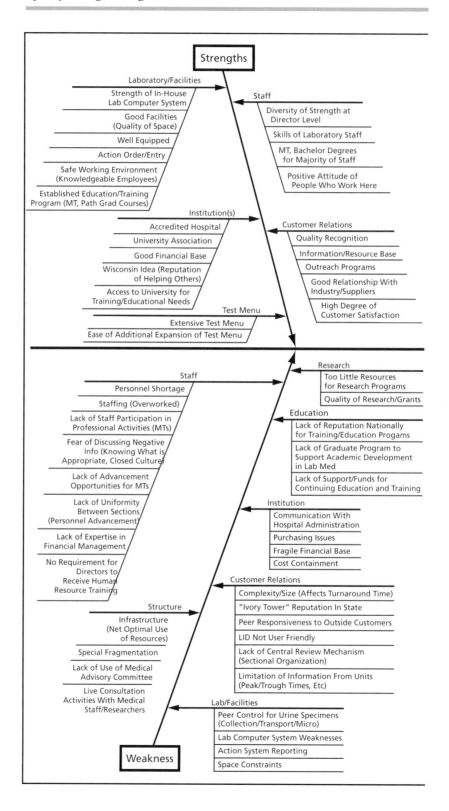

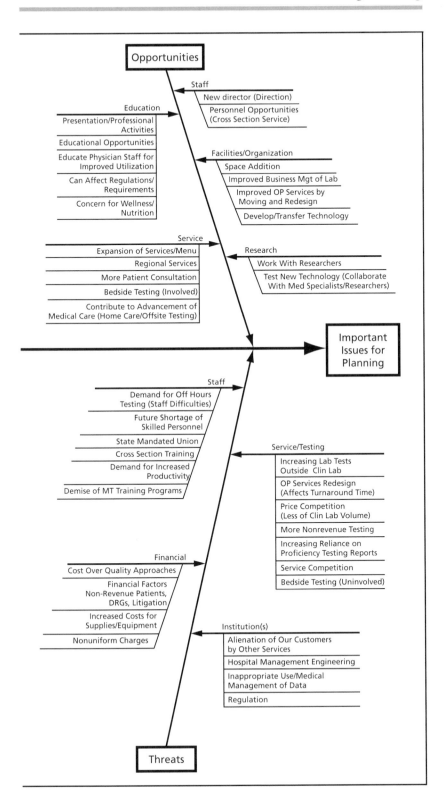

Opportunities

Staff
New director (Direction)
Personnel Opportunities
(Cross Section Service)

Education
Presentation/Professional
Activities
Educational Opportunities
Educate Physician Staff for
Improved Utilization
Can Affect Regulations/
Requirements
Concern for Wellness/
Nutrition

Facilities/Organization
Space Addition
Improved Business Mgt of Lab
Improved OP Services by
Moving and Redesign
Develop/Transfer Technology

Service
Expansion of Services/Menu
Regional Services
More Patient Consultation
Bedside Testing (Involved)
Contribute to Advancement of
Medical Care (Home Care/Offsite Testing)

Research
Work With Researchers
Test New Technology (Collaborate
With Med Specialists/Researchers)

Important
Issues for
Planning

Staff
Demand for Off Hours
Testing (Staff Difficulties)
Future Shortage of
Skilled Personnel
State Mandated Union
Cross Section Training
Demand for Increased
Productivity
Demise of MT Training Programs

Service/Testing
Increasing Lab Tests
Outside Clin Lab
OP Services Redesign
(Affects Turnaround Time)
Price Competition
(Less of Clin Lab Volume)
More Nonrevenue Testing
Increasing Reliance on
Proficiency Testing Reports
Service Competition
Bedside Testing (Uninvolved)

Financial
Cost Over Quality Approaches
Financial Factors
Non-Revenue Patients,
DRGs, Litigation
Increased Costs for
Supplies/Equipment
Nonuniform Charges

Institution(s)
Alienation of Our Customers
by Other Services
Hospital Management Engineering
Inappropriate Use/Medical
Management of Data
Regulation

Threats

Figure 1-10.
Mission statement
from the laboratory.

The University of Wisconsin-Madison's primary mission is to provide an environment in which faculty and students can discover, examine critically, preserve and transmit the knowledge, wisdom and values that help insure the survival of present and future generations with improved quality of life.

As a major component of the University of Wisconsin Center for Health Sciences, the Clinical Laboratories and the Division of Laboratory Medicine strive to be a recognized leader in laboratory medicine by:

- *providing high quality and creative academic programs for health care professionals;*

- *generating new knowledge to provide a foundation for meeting the health care needs of society;*

- *maintaining excellence in service to patients and health care providers, including physicians, nurses, and other health care professionals; and*

- *promoting health care for the residents of the State of Wisconsin.*

Developing Goals and Objectives

The mission statement consists of four elements:

1. Provide high quality and creative academic programs for health care professionals

2. Generate new knowledge to provide a foundation for meeting the health care needs of society

3. Maintain excellence in service to patients and health care providers, including physicians, nurses, and other health care professionals

4. Promote health care for the residents of the State of Wisconsin.

We moved to implement these elements by developing specific goals, objectives, and strategies.

We distributed examples from other organizations, including the American Association for Clinical Chemistry and the Academy for Clinical Laboratory Physicians and Scientists. The committee chair asked each member to take a few minutes to suggest goals for the first element in the mission statement. These were discussed to help clarify the definition of "goals." Committee members were assigned "homework," ie, to write five to seven goals for each of the mission elements for presentation and discussion at the next session. For this exercise, we valued the reflective thinking required for nominal group technique over the spontaneity of brainstorming.

The team presented the goals in a round-robin manner, with each member contributing one goal per turn. The goals were clarified, combined, or separated as needed. We identified 19 goals to support our missions. We also identified several specific objectives for each of these goals. The mission statement and goals/objectives were distributed and clarified to all the laboratory's managers and supervisors. To set priorities for the goals and begin to obtain wider managerial/supervisor "buy-in," we asked each person to "vote," ie, to rate the priority of each goal as high (two points), medium (one point), or low (no points). The Pareto chart in Figure 1–11 summarizes our priorities. Figure 1–12 gives the specific objectives listed under the nine goals with the highest priority.

We developed a mission statement based on analysis of current and future needs and identified goals and objectives that would support those missions. Our next step was to implement the specific objectives. We continued our TQM approach by appointing quality improvement process teams to be guided by a quality improvement planning team.

Implement these elements by developing specific goals, objectives, and strategies.

We continued our TQM approach by appointing quality improvement process teams to be guided by a quality improvement planning team.

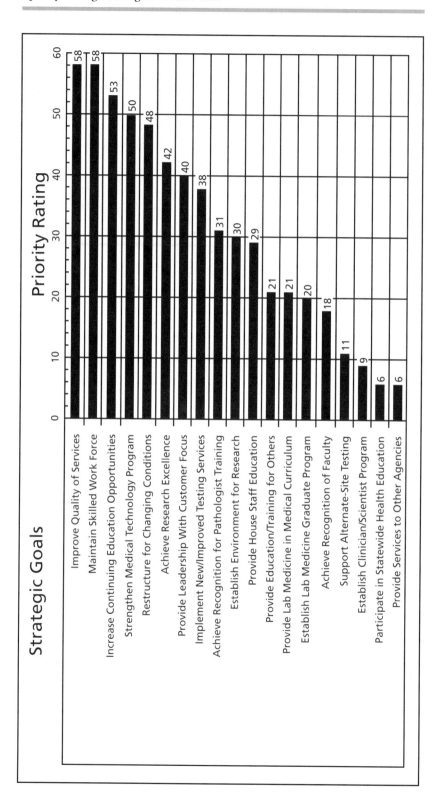

Figure 1-11.
Pareto diagram of priority goals (from *CLMR*. 1991;5:368, with permission).

Goal 1   Achieve national recognition for leadership in quality of laboratory testing services

  Obj 1   Develop multiple cooperative working relationships with users and customers to provide open communication, to obtain a clear understanding of their changing needs, and to help define optimal approaches

  Obj 2   Define quality requirements based on the needs of user or customers to clearly specify the performance to be achieved by laboratory processes

  Obj 3   Maintain quality control and quality assurance programs that provide effective monitors of service and ensure that quality requirements are met

  Obj 4   Establish a quality improvement process to support continuous improvement in testing services

  Obj 5   Establish in-service programs to support quality improvement

Goal 2   Maintain a highly skilled work force to meet the changing needs of users and customers

  Obj 1   Achieve a quality of worklife that supports the needs of the laboratory staff and enhances retention

  Obj 2   Provide a safe work environment

  Obj 3   Achieve higher visibility and recognition for contributions of laboratory personnel

  Obj 4   Develop strategies for recruitment of new personnel

  Obj 5   Develop an education and training program that supports continued development and advancement of a skilled workforce

Goal 3   Increase continuing education opportunities for laboratory personnel

  Obj 1   Establish a formal continuing education program with regular schedule of seminars and workshops to provide on-site opportunities for continuing education

  Obj 2   Provide appropriate resources to attend continuing education programs off-site

  Obj 3   Provide support for presenting continuing education programs for other laboratory personnel

Goal 4   Strengthen the Medical Technology program

  Obj 1   Support student recruitment and clinical training

  Obj 2   Encourage participation of Medical Technologists in professional groups and organizations

Goal 5   Restructure to adapt to the rapidly changing conditions of the health care marketplace

  Obj 1   Adopt organizational strategies and plans to improve flexibility and speed of response

Figure 1-12.
Goals and objectives of laboratory.

Obj 2   Develop staffing strategies and plans to adapt to the changing supply of Medical Technologists

Goal 6   Achieve recognition for the Division of Laboratory Medicine as a center of research excellence in selected areas of study

Obj 1   Have each faculty member engaged in some aspect of basic and/or applied research

Obj 2   Encourage participation of each house officer/fellow in Pathology and Laboratory Medicine in some aspect of applied and/or basic research

Obj 3   Engage graduate students, post-doctoral fellows, MD fellows/clinicians, and other scientists associated with the Division or working actively in research under the guidance of Division faculty

Obj 4   Provide opportunities for Medical Technologists and other classified staff with interest in and aptitude for collaborative research with faculty

Obj 5   Provide research opportunities in Pathology and Laboratory Medicine for MD/PhD candidates

Obj 6   Encourage collaborative research with members of other departments

Obj 7   Disseminate information generated by this research activity widely via publications in scientific and professional journals, presentations at scientific meetings, and sponsorship of scientific conferences

Obj 8   Increase research grants and contracts within the Division

Goal 7   Provide management leadership that focuses on the changing needs of internal and external users and customers

Obj 1   Establish a complement of directors, consultants, managers, supervisors, and technical specialists to provide leadership in development, improvement, and management of testing services

Obj 2   Develop direct patient consultative services to enhance the use of laboratory services and data and to support the changing needs of users

Obj 3   Provide effective, open communication with internal and external users and customers, including laboratory personnel at all levels

Obj 4   Establish planning activities to help solve problems and maximize opportunities in the future

Goal 8   Implement new and improved testing services to meet the changing needs of users and customers

Obj 1   Expand the testing menu to satisfy changing needs of users and customers

Obj 2   Expand and improve services for outpatients and outside clients

Figure 1-12 (cont.)

Obj 3   Utilize newly developing technology, such as bar coding, to expand testing services and improve productivity

Obj 4   Improve the cost-effectiveness, productivity, and appropriate utilization of testing processes to satisfy the changing reimbursement policies

Obj 5   Facilitate appropriate test ordering and interpretation to support rapid introduction and changes of testing services

Obj 6   Develop forms of data representation that are easier for physicians to understand and facilitate the implementation and application of testing services

Goal 9   Become nationally recognized for excellence in training of practicing pathologists in Laboratory Medicine

Obj 1   Improve residency training in Laboratory Medicine

LESSONS LEARNED

The long-range planning team's work was indispensable to the change program. Some of its accomplishments are as follows:

1. The reason for change was introduced and acceptance of change begun.

2. The concept of TQM was introduced to the laboratory director and to many laboratory employees.

3. TQM tools were taught and used.

4. A mission statement, goals, and objectives were developed and accepted.

5. A direction was set and a style of management introduced.

6. Many laboratory personnel gained experience in these processes.

7. Strategic goals and objectives were implemented.

There are several critical elements that contributed to the long-range planning team's success. The director of quality assurance had knowledge of and experience in TQM. The manager of quality assurance was a trained facilitator and was vital to the success of the project. Although our facilitator came from our own organization, this is not a requirement for success.

The QA director was a longtime laboratory employee and had considerable experience and insight to help select the composition of the team. He also had the respect and trust of other employees.

There are several critical elements that contributed to the long-range planning team's success.

Laboratorians deal in numbers and have some understanding of statistics, quality control, control charts, etc. They use the scientific method daily. These factors resulted in a short TQM learning curve for most of the team members.

The project had the strong support of the new laboratory director, ie, upper management.

The team chair set and held to an action line with deadlines for completion of each task.

In retrospect, there were some things that we might have improved. The goals probably would have been easier to implement if the team membership had included a senior hospital administrator and a senior representative from the medical school or academic department of pathology. We had asked for representation from hospital administration and from the academic department; however, hospital administration appointed a junior member who eventually left the full-time employ of the hospital. The academic department chose not to appoint anyone. The medical school, ie, dean's office, was not approached. Consequently, the absence of representatives from senior hospital administration and the academic department had the positive effect of allowing us to focus on the laboratory per se; however, their absence precluded hearing from others with perhaps different perspectives. Further, it was exactly those two elements that would eventually be needed to implement change fully. Nonetheless, the long-range planning teams accomplished all its immediate goals and did so in 3 months.

REFERENCES

1. US Dept of Health and Human Services. Medicare, Medicaid, and CLIA Programs; regulations implementing the Clinical Laboratory Improvement Amendments of 1988 (CLIA). Final rule. *Federal Register.* February 28, 1992;57:7002–7186.

2. Deming WE. *Quality, Productivity, and Competitive Position.* Cambridge, Mass: Massachusetts Institute of Technology, Center for Advanced Study; 1982.

3. Deming WE. *Out of the Crisis.* Cambridge, Mass: Massachusetts Institute of Technology, Center for Advanced Study; 1987.

4. Hammer M, Champy J. *Reengineering the Corporation.* New York: Harper Business; 1993.

5. Juran JM. The quality trilogy. *Quality Progress.* August 1986:19–24.

6. Juran JM, Endres A. *Quality Improvement for Services.* Wilton, Conn: Juran Institute, Inc; 1986.

7. Juran JM. *Planning for Quality.* New York, NY: The Free Press; 1988.

8. Westgard JO, Barry PL. *Cost-Effective Quality Control: Managing the Quality and Productivity of Analytical Processes.* Washington, DC: AACC Press; 1986: 1–32.

9. Eggert AA, Westgard JO, Barry PL, Blankenheim TJ, Emmerich KA, Becker DJ. Automated collection and analysis of turnaround time data from a clinical laboratory computer system. *Informatics in Pathology.* 1987;2:5–14.

10. Koch DD, Oryall JJ, Quam EF, et al. Selection of medically useful QC procedures for individual tests on a multi-test analytical system. *Clin Chem.* 1990;36:230–233.

11. Westgard JO, Barry PL. Total quality control: evolution of quality systems in health care laboratories. *Lab Med.* 1989;20:377–384.

12. Westgard JO, Burnett RW, Bowers GN. Quality management science in clinical chemistry: a dynamic framework for continuous improvement. *Clin Chem.* 1990;36:1712–1716.

13. Westgard JO, Barry PL. Beyond quality assurance: committing to quality improvement. *Lab Med.* 1989;20:241–247.

14. Westgard JO, Barry PL, Tomar RH. Implementing total quality management (TQM) in health care laboratories. *CLMR.* 1991;5:353–370.

15. Holmberg SR. Strategic planning: a management tool for the clinical laboratory. *CLMR.* 1988;2:185–194.

16. Folger JC. The business plan. *CLMR.* 1988;2:31–34.

17. Morrisey GL. Who Needs a Mission Statement? You Do. *Training and Development Journal.* March 1988: 50–52.

Total Quality Management

Developing Process Focus and Team Skills

COMMITTING TO TOTAL QUALITY MANAGEMENT

The development of a new strategic plan by the project team approach gave us direction for the future. Next, we needed a way to implement the plan. Based on our team's experience, we decided to use the project-by-project approach as the methodology for implementation. The implementation effort was guided by a quality steering team (QST) that was responsible for identifying doable projects, defining the mission of each project, selecting team members, establishing rules and responsibilities, providing trained facilitators, and supporting team training. The QST had as members the laboratory director, the senior laboratory manager, the associate director and the supervisor for quality assurance, the associate director for administration, and the manager of data processing. We recognized that all projects seemed to require computer support for data collection, thus establishing the importance of computer and data processing support to establish baseline measures and document process improvements.

We decided to use the project-by-project approach as the methodology for implementation.

Initial projects were guided by the strategic plan and focused on an employee survey for consensus on laboratory goals, continuing education for laboratory employees, recruitment and retention of personnel, development of a plan for laboratory space, consolidation of special chemistry services (which turned out to be a precursor to our reengineering efforts), preparation of a laboratory test ordering handbook, improvement of patient reports, and improvement of customer services, with special attention to telephone communications and services.

In carrying out these projects, the QST developed in-house training materials to support the new teams. These materials were also used to present several workshops on "Caring for Quality" at state and national professional meetings. Approximately 30% of our staff received training during this time. In addition, outside training for team facilitation was provided by a State of Wisconsin 10-day course for three of our medical technologists who served as facilitators for these project teams.

Most of these projects took longer and were more difficult to complete than was anticipated, which again pointed to the need for careful selection of projects, adherence to a systematic team process and problem-solving model, careful selection of team members, management commitment for implementation of recommendations, a higher level of support and tools for planning projects, ongoing team and facilitator training, and the need for improved management of projects. Among our section directors and laboratory managers and supervisors, there was also a concern for the amount of time being spent in team meetings, particularly those teams whose members had little experience from earlier pilot projects. Team recommendations for changes also ran into some opposition from managers and supervisors who were not involved in the team process. Consequently, the authority of the traditional management structure began to be challenged by the team process. We came to understand that total quality management (TQM) was not confined to narrower issues of quality but involved the entire laboratory and everything that was being done. We discovered that this process was empowering to some people and threatening to others. TQM was being taken seriously by our staff, whether they were for it or against it.

With each round of new projects, we gained experience, trained more of our personnel in simple problem-solving tools and techniques, and became more effective in carrying out the projects. Most gratifyingly, we began to see the team problem-solving process and tools being used informally, without the need for a facilitator and without the authorization of a formal team. Many employees were able to solve problems and improve the laboratory without formal intervention by management. This was a significant accomplishment for TQM in our laboratory and allowed us to start thinking about the next stages of process improvement.

ADOPTING THE GOAL/QPC MODEL FOR TQM

Several new faculty, directors, and managers had joined our staff and needed to be introduced to TQM; thus, there was the need to provide a new round of training to maintain our momentum and continue our progress. By the fall of 1991, good training materials were available, and we decided to adopt the approach being developed by GOAL/QPC, a nonprofit organization in Methuen, Mass, that helps companies improve its quality, productivity, and competitiveness (QPC). We were impressed by GOAL's scholarly yet practical orientation, as revealed in its research report "Total Quality Management Master Plan: An Implementation Strategy."[1] We were also interested in its training materials for the seven management and planning tools that were better-suited to management problems and applications than other programs aimed at classical indus-

The authority of the traditional management structure began to be challenged by the team process.

TQM was not confined to narrower issues of quality but involved the entire laboratory.

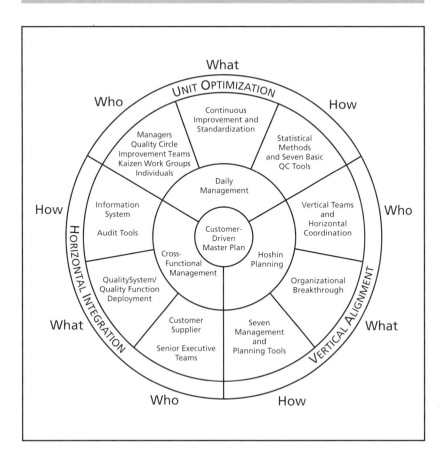

Figure 2-1.
GOAL/QPC TQM Wheel (with permission from GOAL/QPC, Methuen, MA 01844).

trial processes. The need for a higher level of planning and better tools to support planning was one of the most important lessons we had learned. We took advantage of all the resources GOAL provided, including workshops, video training programs, and written materials. We also legitimized our approach and efforts by aligning them with emerging plans and approaches from business and industry. At this point, we were advancing beyond the traditional quality management practices used in our hospital and in health care laboratories in general.

The GOAL model for TQM is shown in Figure 2-1 in the form of a wheel. This type of diagram is read from the center out. The central emphasis is a customer-driven master plan, whose goals and objectives are accomplished by the three systems or mechanisms identified as (1) daily management, (2) Hoshin planning, and (3) cross-functional management. In our evolving approach, project teams and individual problem solving provided the daily management mechanism, and our strategic quality planning was the impetus for Hoshin planning. We

There was a need for a higher level of planning and better tools to support planning.

viewed cross-functional management in the context of our hospital organization and identified aspects that we could partially implement on our own, but found that this organizationwide mechanism would be limited by the hospital's slow acceptance of cross-departmental teams and the replacement of traditional committees with a team problem-solving process. Each of these mechanisms uses certain tools and techniques, as identified in the next outer ring of the figure. Together these efforts lead to unit optimization, vertical alignment, and horizontal integration, as shown in the outermost ring.

The GOAL implementation plan identified a 10-step process.

The GOAL implementation plan identified a 10-step process, as shown in Figure 2-2. A decision to implement TQM (step 1) leads to an examination of customer needs (step 2) and the critical processes (step 3) for meeting those needs. Initial teams (step 4) provide experience in quality improvement methodology and an understanding of the quality improvement process. With this background, a 5-year plan (step 5) can be developed to guide the next stage of implementation (steps 6 through 10). Because of our past efforts to implement TQM, we believed that we had done much of the work in steps 1 through 4 and needed to develop the plan called for in step 5. We were experiencing the problem of managing momentum (step 6) and needed to develop better planning approaches (step 7) and increase the involvement of individuals in daily management (step 8). New teams (step 9) would continue to be important, but by now we had a significant bit of team experience. Evaluating progress (step 10) is a difficult and ongoing problem.

TRAINING FACULTY AND DIRECTORS

In January 1992, we began a new training course for our faculty and directors, which included the hospital administrator responsible for the laboratory area. The objectives of the course, as developed by QST, are shown in Table 2-1. Each participant was provided a copy of the GOAL research report to provide a general background for the course. The training began with a half-day retreat and continued with 9 weekly sessions of 1 to 2 hours each. The general format focused on the specific objectives for each session, provided a brief review of the previous session, introduced each topic with a 20 to 30 minute segment from the GOAL/QPC video training program, used problems and exercises to apply the concepts, and discussed specific applications in our laboratory. The leader and facilitator roles for each session were rotated among the QST members and one other trained facilitator.

TQM Decision (Session 1)

The opening training session provided a review of TQM principles and practices Deming's plan, do, check, act (PDCA) cycle Juran's quality

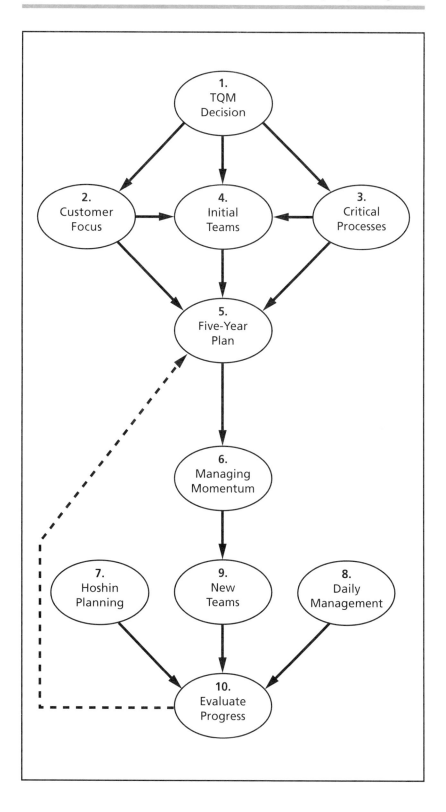

Figure 2-2
GOAL/QPC 10-element model for TQM implementation (with permission from GOAL/QPC, Methuen, MA 01844).

Table 2-1.

TRAINING OBJECTIVES FOR **TQM** IMPLEMENTATION COURSE FOR LABORATORY FACULTY AND DIRECTORS

Overview

1. Review the background of the development and implementation of TQM
2. Understand the four major components that are integrated into the GOAL/QPC model for TQM
3. Understand the 10 elements or steps in the GOAL/QPC implementation plan
4. Identify activities for the second phase of TQM implementation at University of Wisconsin division of laboratory medicine

Top management's decision to implement TQM

1. Review University of Wisconsin interest and support for TQM
2. Discuss potential benefits and likely problems in implementing TQM
3. Understand interest and commitment of University of Wisconsin division of laboratory medicine
4. Review role of Quality Steering Team in supporting TQM implementation

Understanding the customer

1. Review assessment of customers and customer needs from laboratory strategic plan
2. Identify baseline measures of laboratory performance
3. Introduce the concept of Quality Function Deployment (QFD)
4. Illustrate QFD by determination of operating specifications for precision, accuracy, and QC based on analytical quality requirements, such as CLIA PT criteria
5. Discuss role of laboratory medical advisory committee

Identify and evaluate critical processes

1. Describe the main processes of the division of laboratory medicine
2. Identify the three to five processes that are most critical in your own management position
3. Generalize the most critical processes for this level of management
4. Identify the customers of those critical processes
5. Identify the requirements for satisfying those customers

Initial pilot project teams

1. Review the management agenda (from the strategic plan) for activities of project teams in the division of laboratory medicine
2. Review the problem solving model and tools being used by project teams
3. Summarize "lessons learned" from initial project teams

4.Discuss benefits and difficulties with project teams

Table 2-1, continued

5. Clarify role of faculty and directors in relation to project team activities

Assess organization and create 5-year plan

1. Review our current strategic plan

2. Review laboratory mission and values statement

3. Clarify laboratory vision

4. Identify two to three breakthrough objectives for the next year

5. Discuss a mechanism for breakthrough planning for 3- to 5-year time-frame

Managing TQM momentum

1. Discuss mechanisms for recognition of employees for team and individual contributions and accomplishments

2. Review current QST efforts for improving the quality improvement process

3. Identify opportunities for expanding TQM in daily process management

4. Identify training needs for expanded implementation of TQM

5. Identify other resources (facilitators, etc) needed for supporting expanded TQM activities

Achieving breakthrough objectives through Hoshin planning

1. Review and clarify departmental breakthrough objectives for this year

2. Identify section objectives that align with laboratory objectives

3. Determine measurements to monitor achievement of section objectives

4. Discuss possible problems or obstacles in achieving this year's breakthrough objectives

Daily management and standardization

1. Review critical process methodology as an approach for integrating TQM into the work of each individual

2. Discuss empowerment and ownership of critical processes for section managers, supervisors, analysts, etc

3. Identify driving and restraining forces that affect our ability to implement daily process management

4. Establish section objectives for implementation of daily process management

5. Discuss how employee performance evaluations could be modified to be more consistent with TQM principles

New functional and cross-functional teams

1. Understand the purpose of functional and cross-functional management

Table 2-1, continued

2. Identify existing cross-functional mechanisms in the division of laboratory medicine

3. Identify additional activities that are needed for cross-functional management

Review TQM progress and revise 5-year plan

1. Discuss need for 5-year customer driven master plan

2. Identify mechanisms for updating the laboratory strategic plan to provide the 5-year master plan

3. Establish a timetable for development of the 5-year master plan

TQM = Total Quality Management; QPC = quality, productivity, and competitiveness; QC = Quality Control; PT = Proficiency Testing; QST = quality steering team.

trilogy; and our integration of these industrial models to form our 5-Q model for laboratory quality management. We emphasized that this 5-Q model provided a scientific management process that was applicable to all of us in our management and individual work processes. We took advantage of the national attention and recognition being achieved by a couple of local quality consultants, Brian Joiner and Peter Scholtes, to further clarify this process orientation through their description of TQM:

Simply put, total quality management is an approach to management which focuses on giving top value to customers.

"Simply put, total quality management is an approach to management which focuses on giving top value to customers by building excellence into every aspect of the organization. This is done by creating an environment which allows and encourages everyone to contribute to the organization and by developing skills which enable them to study scientifically and constantly improve every process by which work is accomplished. In total quality management, the emphasis is on studying processes and executing them better and better to provide customers with products and services of every increasing value at lower cost."

This upside-down organization chart was intended to challenge the control style of management.

With this emphasis on processes, we then presented a view of the organization as a *system of processes supported by management,* as shown in Figure 2-3. This upside-down organization chart was intended to challenge the military control model of management that was most familiar to our faculty and directors and is typical of the control style of man-

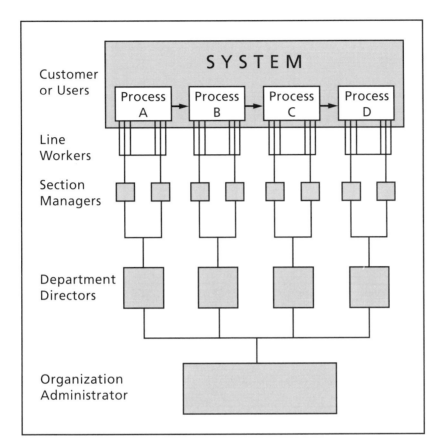

Customer or Users

SYSTEM

| Process A | Process B | Process C | Process D |

Line Workers

Section Managers

Department Directors

Organization Administrator

Figure 2-3.
TQM view of an orga-
nization as a system of
processes supported by
management.

agement in most health care organizations. In the upside–down organi-zation chart, lineworkers or our bench-level analysts become the important players because they are involved in those work processes that directly affect the patients, customers, or users of laboratory services. Managers, directors, and administrators are further away and have less of a direct impact on the immediate delivery of services and satisfaction of patients and customers. We included a brainstorming exercise in this opening session for the faculty to express and discuss their thoughts and ideas on the guiding principles of TQM.

We next pointed out that TQM was a specific issue in the new Joint Commission on Accreditation of Healthcare Organizations (JCAHO) standards (called continuous quality improvement). We believed that there would be a need for more widespread implementa-tion of TQM in our laboratory and hospital. Concerns were raised about the lack of resources, lack of hospital activity, and lack of time.

The hospital administrator indicated that administration was supportive of department efforts to achieve TQM, but was not likely to take the lead. Hospital administration was studying approaches taken at other university hospitals, such as the University of Michigan, that had made a commitment to aggressive, hospital-wide implementation. In spite of the hospital's reticence, the presence of a hospital administrator in these training sessions added a new dimension because most of the laboratory employees had little previous contact with upper hospital management. Having gained the faculty's attention, it was time for more detailed discussions of the GOAL 10-step implementation plan, which was the basis for the rest of the training sessions.

Customer Focus (Session 2)

The purpose of this session was to ensure that our TQM efforts would be focused on the needs of the customers. Customers of laboratory services include external customers such as the physicians and nurses who order the tests and the patients who are the ultimate beneficiaries of laboratory services, as well as the agencies and organizations who pay for the tests. In addition, laboratory sections are often the internal customers of each other. Phlebotomy and sample processing sections provided good examples for illustrating how their services are also focused on the needs of the analytical sections of the laboratory.

In understanding customers' perceptions of quality, three different classes were discussed. The first class is *one-dimensional quality* which involves attributes that are directly related to customer satisfaction. Better fulfillment of the quality requirement leads to improved customer satisfaction. A nonlaboratory example might be a food service where faster service and better tasting food leads to greater customer satisfaction. In the laboratory, we also expect that quicker turnaround and an extensive test menu lead to greater satisfaction of the physicians, nurses, and ultimately patients. The second class is *expected quality,* which are attributes that are often assumed or taken for granted. Nobody notices when the requirement is satisfied, but customers will be unhappy if it is not satisfied. A nonlaboratory example is airline safety, which is assumed and expected by all passengers but does not provide any special satisfaction. In the laboratory, analytical quality is expected. All our customers assume that the test results are reliable. There is no extra customer satisfaction gained from providing accurate test results, but there would be great dissatisfaction and anger, and possibly legal action, if an error occurred. The third type of attribute is *exciting quality,* so-named because it is unexpected. A nonlaboratory example involves a local pizza restaurant that had a drive-through window, where the employees would often wash the windshields of the cars while the customers were waiting to get their pizza. In the laboratory, an exciting quality might be when the phlebotomists remember the names of the patients and are able to address them personally whenever they see them. Initially, new diagnostic services that are made available often invoke a sense of unexpected quality from health care providers.

The industrial technique of quality function deployment (QFD) was also introduced during this session to illustrate a systematic process for translating customer needs into quality requirements, process characteristics, process specifications, and control procedures. One important message was that customers cannot directly tell us the process specifications that we should use. For example, most laboratorians have received calls from physicians who demand faster performance of the tests they have ordered. If we listen directly to the customer and go into the laboratory, we may be able to reduce the testing time perhaps by 50%, from 12 to 6 minutes; however, the real problem may be that the transport of the specimen is taking 60 minutes. Consequently, reducing our test performance time by 6 minutes will have little impact on the assay turnaround time. Therefore, even though we did respond as the customer demanded, we did not address the real issue.

Translating customer needs into quality requirements.

Another example is that physicians do not really know what precision and accuracy is needed for laboratory tests. Physicians can tell us how they use and interpret laboratory data, but the laboratory must translate those needs into quality requirements (eg, clinical decision interval, allowable analytical total error), precision and accuracy specifications (Coefficient of Variance and bias), and quality control procedures (control rules, number of control measurements). Given that analytical quality is an expected characteristic and that the laboratory will need to take complete responsibility for ensuring the quality of its tests, it should be an important part of TQM to develop clinical and analytical quality requirements for every test. The laboratory then would translate those requirements into operating specifications for precision, accuracy, and quality control. We have implemented quality functional deployment in a variety of ways: (1) the development of quality-planning models[2-3]; (2) new tools such as the chart of operating specifications (OPSpecs chart)[4-5]; and (3) new technology for analytical quality management in the form of computer software.[6] The latter translates analytical or clinical quality requirements into operating specifications and provides automatic selection of quality control (QC) procedures on the basis of the defined quality requirement for the test and the observed imprecision and inaccuracy of the test method. Thus the industrial concept of QFD has a practical application for every test in every laboratory.

Physicians do not really know what precision and accuracy is needed for laboratory tests . . . . the laboratory must translate those needs into quality requirements.

Critical Processes for Laboratory Service and Management (Session 3)

Any repeated work activity is a process.

Any repeated work activity is a *process;* thus, virtually all that is accomplished in a laboratory and a health care organization comes about through processes. Processes may be divided into steps that often become *subprocesses* that involve individuals performing a few special operations or procedures. Processes can be combined into *systems* that define the larger operations of the organizations where sections or departments are linked together to provide services to customers and patients.

Processes can be combined into systems that define the larger operations of the organizations.

Two flowcharting techniques are commonly used to describe processes. The first is a top-down flowchart that is used to map out broadly the flow of a process by identifying the major steps (across the top of a page) and then their substeps (as a list under each of the major steps), as shown in Figure 2-4, for the process of implementing TQM. A detailed flowchart makes use of a standard set of symbols that describe the steps, logic, and loops of a process, such as shown in Figure 2-5, which describes our process of handling mislabeled specimens and illustrates the complexity that gets added to accommodate exceptions. In flowcharting, we have found it useful to have additional symbols for a "brick wall," a "black hole," and "magic happens" to describe initially ill-defined processes and identify those areas that need to be refined. The detailed flowchart is technically more difficult and time-consuming to construct, but is advantageous because it describes the logic for decision-making steps in the process and identifies loops in the process. Loops should be eliminated whenever possible to reduce complexity and improve efficiency.

Useful to have additional symbols for a "brick wall," a "black hole," and "magic happens."

Even with newer and more sophisticated PC computer programs for flowcharting, it still takes considerable time and effort to define a process. Regardless how simple the process, it is always interesting to see how differently members of a group view the process and the steps they are actually performing. Just the attempt to write down the process and gain consensus on what is being done is often a big step in standardizing and improving how work gets done. Clinical decision making and medical practice are even more complicated, which is why critical pathways are so difficult to develop and yet are so essential for improving medical practice.

Key to understanding and managing processes is the identification of customers and their requirements and the recognition of the responsibility of the supplier to satisfy those customer requirements. Suppliers also may need to deal with both external and internal customers, eg, phlebotomy acquires specimens to satisfy the orders of physicians (external customer) and needs of patients (external consumer), then delivers those specimens to the laboratory (internal customer) for analysis. The

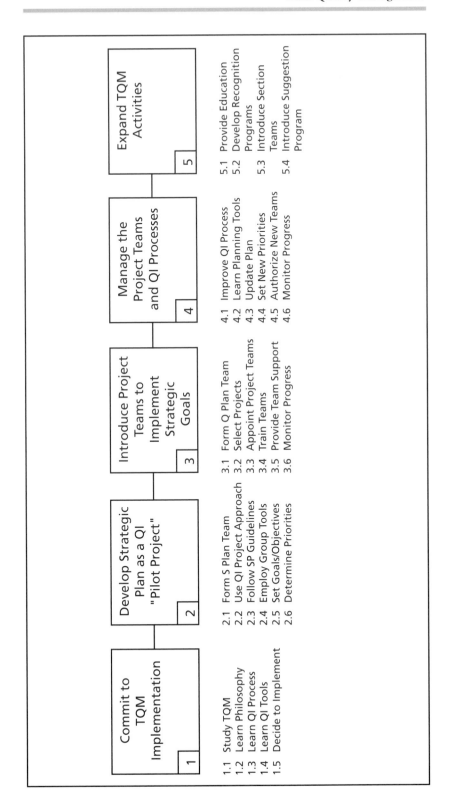

Figure 2-4.
Example top-down flowchart for implementing TQM. TQM = total quality management; QI = quality improvement; SP = strategic plan.

Figure 2-5.
Example of detailed
flowchart for process
of handling mislabeled
specimens.

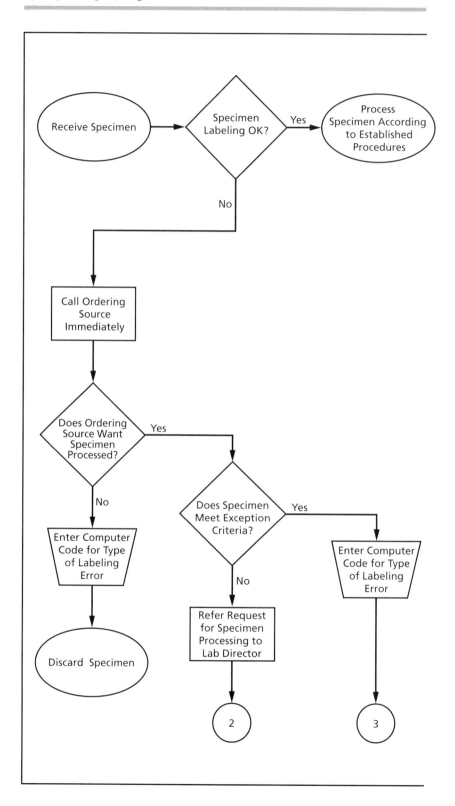

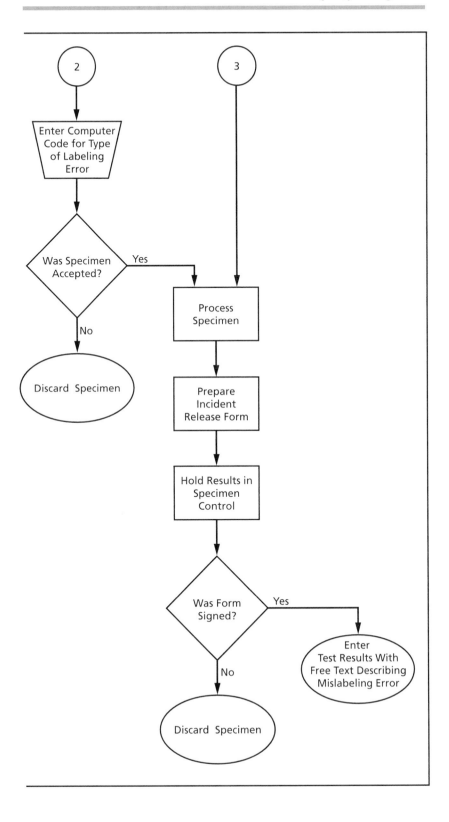

The quality of a service depends on identifying the customers and satis-fying their needs.

Customer-supplier interactions are two-way streets.

quality of a service depends on identifying all these customers and satis-fying their needs. Often organizations focus on external customers, without adequately considering internal customers, which usually leads to unhappy employees and, eventually, to unhappy customers.

Virtually all customer-supplier interactions are two-way streets, ie, purchasing needs to acquire materials with the proper specifications to satisfy the needs of laboratory analysts, but laboratory analysts need to identify their needs properly through specifications that can be used to acquire the appropriate materials. In our operation, these internal types of customer-supplier interactions have been troublesome, sometimes tense, and occasionally heated. Our purchasing department, for example, also must be concerned about satisfying the requirements of the State of Wisconsin, which emphasizes the use of competitive bids to achieve the lowest prices. This often results in changing vendors and getting new products or materials that require considerable in-house testing by the laboratory, which increases laboratory costs of operation, even if the prices are cheaper. We have often found it difficult to adapt our internal bureaucracy, improve these internal customer relationships, and develop the teamwork necessary to improve internal processes.

It is essential in the beginning to focus on the most important processes, or critical *processes.*

Because there are so many processes that are in use by any organi-zation, it is essential in the beginning to focus on the most important processes, or *critical processes*. One idea is to think about the *main event*. What are we really in business for anyway? In the laboratory, the main event has to do with producing test results. The important steps of the main event involve the ordering of laboratory tests, preparation of patients, obtaining specimens from patients, transporting those speci-mens to the laboratory, analyzing the specimens for the appropriate tests, reporting those test results and interpretation, then documenting the process for future reference (and, of course, billing for fees and col-lecting the money, which are usually considered so important those steps are taken over directly by the hospital or health care organization).

In discussing critical processes, we introduced a methodology for analysis and assessment based on guidelines from Mark Finster, PhD, a professor in the Business School at University of Wisconsin-Madison. The steps involve (1) identifying a critical process, (2) identifying the main products or services of this process, (3) identifying the customers (end user, next process or internal customer, others), (4) identifying the high priority customers, (5) identifying the needs of the high priority customer, (6) identifying the three highest priority needs, (7) identifying the key quality features or characteristics related to those needs, (8) pri-oritizing the relationship between customer needs and quality charac-teristics as strong/major, normal/definite, or possible/minor, (9) defining performance specifications for those key quality characteristics,

(10) identifying measures and monitors for controlling the performance of these key characteristics, (11) identifying current or baseline performance, and (12) identifying opportunities for process improvement.

The concept of critical processes is important to everyone because every person in the laboratory can view his or her work in terms of managing a few critical processes. The types of processes differ at various levels of the organization, but everyone needs to know what his or her critical processes are and how they should be assessed and managed. In this way, the job of every single person in the laboratory can benefit from the process assessment and improvement methodology.

Every person can view his or her work in terms of managing a few critical processes.

Brainstorming by the faculty and section directors identified several critical processes that are important for this level of management, such as: forecasting test volumes and future service needs, planning and prioritizing laboratory activities, selecting appropriate services to be offered, setting test specifications, developing new products and services, allocating resources, selecting and evaluating personnel, and facilitating personnel transactions. Discussion of these processes helped clarify the service responsibilities of faculty and section directors and made it easier to differentiate the responsibilities of managers and supervisors.

Reviewing Project Team Experience (Session 4)

TQM and quality improvement methodology were new ideas to some of our new faculty and section directors who were not experienced in the laboratory's quality improvement. We needed to educate and gain support from the new group and reaffirm commitment from the rest of middle management. Potential conflicts between project teams and the existing management structure needed to be recognized and discussed as we continued our transition to a "quality" organization.

In our laboratory, a project team was composed of a leader, facilitator, adviser (optional), and members who were supported by top management including the QST, our supervisors and managers. The QST was responsible for identifying issues; selecting the project; writing the initial mission statement; establishing a timetable if needed; selecting the team leader, facilitator, and team members; and providing the necessary training. The QST met regularly to provide guidance (refine the mission statement), facilitate system changes to accommodate project work (data gathering), allocate new resources when needed (data processing support), clear organization barriers (help team members attend meetings if time demands conflicted with section responsibilities), and follow up on the implementation of recommendations for improvements (work with administration and management to see that the resources were allocated to support implementation). After completion of a project, QST was responsible for recognizing team efforts and accomplishments, referring implementation to appropriate sections or individuals, and evaluating and improving the team process.

A project team focused on a single problem or issue as defined in its mission statement.

A project team focused on a single problem or issue as defined in its mission statement and was active until its mission was completed. The team leader was usually a manager in the project area because implementation of any changes would require the involvement and commitment of the local managers. The facilitator was usually one of half a dozen of our own technologists who had obtained formal training in quality improvement methodology and facilitation; occasionally we used an outside facilitator who was familiar with laboratory and health care issues. Team members came from different levels within the labora-

Team members came from different levels within the laboratory but were considered to be equals in the team process.

tory but were considered to be equals in the team process. Their essential qualifications were to be knowledgeable about the process; be able to work effectively in a group; be willing to be involved; and have time available from their section, which meant that faculty, directors, and managers had some voice in their participation. Team members were responsible for attending all meetings, performing assignments on time, representing coworkers, recommending agenda items, gathering data, contributing to solutions, establishing monitors to track the effectiveness of improvements, participating in presentations, and critiquing and improving the team process.

Decisions were based on data and guided by the seven step problem-solving methodology.

The team was expected to make its decisions based on data and guided by the seven-step problem-solving methodology that had become standard on the University of Wisconsin campus and the City of Madison:

- Step 1. Define the project. This step involves identifying, prioritizing, and selecting issues suitable for resolution by a project team. A problem statement is written, the project team appointed, resources authorized, and training provided. A prioritization matrix is used as a tool in the selection of issues.

- Step 2. Examine the process. The project team initially outlines the process to be studied, identifies the customers or users of the process, identifies the needs of those customers and users, defines boundaries of the problem, identifies measures of process performance, obtains baseline data, and then reviews and refines the problem statement in light of present knowledge of the process. Flow diagrams can be used to outline the process. A brainstorming session can be used to initially identify customers and their needs. Surveys are developed to get direct customer input. Data from these sources can be organized by fishbone or cause-and-effect diagrams. Checksheets are used to help collect baseline data. An action plan is then developed.

- Step 3. Identify root causes. With the knowledge of the process that has been gained, possible causes are identified and prioritized. Data are collected and analyzed to identify root causes. A Pareto diagram is often used to arrange the causes in order of importance.

- Step 4. Develop improvement. Possible solutions are identified and evaluated to select the best solution. A description of the improved process is prepared. Barriers to change are identified and a plan for pilot implementation is developed. Force-field analysis is used to assess the relative balance of barriers to change and drivers of change.

- Step 5. Verify improvement. A pilot improvement plan is implemented. New performance data are collected and compared with earlier baseline data to verify the improvement. Based on the pilot study, new guidelines are developed for general improvements.

- Step 6. Standardize improvement. The standard process to be implemented is formalized, control measures are identified, an overall implementation plan is developed, the standardized process improvement is implemented, and performance is monitored.

- Step 7. Maximize gains. The project is documented, the quality improvement process itself is evaluated to suggest possible improvements, and the "lessons learned" are identified to document the new knowledge so it can be passed on to others. Other applications of the process improvements are identified, as well as other opportunities for improving the current process. The work of the project team is publicized, contributions of team members are recognized, and the project is concluded.

The support required for these project teams and the team problem-solving process was a topic of considerable discussion because these resources came from the sections themselves. Support requires training, time for members to attend meetings and do their project assignments, facilitator support for planning and team meetings, funding for materials needed in the projects, and support and commitment to implement the improvements.

Assess the Organization and Create a 5-Year Plan (Session 5)
The GOAL/QPC model recommends "Hoshin planning," which is a form of strategic planning that identifies a few key breakthrough areas

Strategic planning identifies a few key breakthrough areas.

that are critical for the success of an organization. Breakthrough areas are then communicated up, down, and across the organization through "catch-ball"—back and forth discussions to clarify the boundaries and identify specific objectives for implementation. This process was similar to what we had been following, ie, providing project teams with mission statements, which were then clarified by back and forth discussions between the project team and the QST. Through catch-ball, every individual develops an understanding of his or her role in achieving the organization's breakthrough objectives.

As examples of breakthrough objectives, our laboratory had earlier placed a priority on the following: establish and expand molecular probe technology, improve basic laboratory systems to increase safety and efficiency and to decrease errors, plan and implement an effective outreach program, increase and improve educational opportunities, increase research capacity, and implement TQM to provide a vehicle for achieving breakthroughs.

In preparation for developing a new plan, we updated our earlier organizational self-assessment to take into account changes in customer needs, regulatory issues, ethical issues, and competitive benchmarks. We also reviewed our earlier mission and values statements and a new rough draft of a vision statement, all of which were considered important in providing direction for the future by understanding the driving forces and the commitment necessary to make organizational changes. Defining a vision is important for helping people understand the higher purpose of the organization, its reason for being, the philosophy behind its daily activities. Vision should guide the organization's planning for the future. In spite of recognizing its importance, the laboratory had a difficult time composing a vision statement that could be embraced by most of the laboratory's employees.

We brainstormed two questions—What do you envision for laboratory medicine in 10 to 15 years? What do we want to become? The future of laboratory medicine was described by the following collection of comments: decentralized, near total automation, consulting role for laboratory personnel rather than doers of tests, self-sufficient in testing, testing for "function", organized by technology, integrated with other medical information, interpretive reports, reduced numbers of tests, closer alignment with customers, different tests (new areas of interest), automation through expert systems, lean organization with less resources, greater reliance on rapid near-patient testing, demand for quickness in service, trend to centralization, direct dealing with the patient for testing, monopolization of test methodology by a few manufacturers, more physician reliance on the computer and the need for data sharing via computer, direct orders and return of results to computer on units, wellness testing for disease prevention, more reliance on computers in general with direct reports to physicians, different external and regulator mechanisms, development of "consortia" based laboratory medicine organizations, fierce competition, and more cost containment.

With a sense of what was to come in laboratory medicine, we turned to the issue of what we want or need to become, again using a brainstorming format to collect the following ideas: develop the next generation data handling capability, customer/client relations department, be more flexible, become consultants, streamline processing for high volume tests, develop more scientific competence and a better understanding of the relationship of tests to patient outcome, reconstruct and rebuild our physical plant, increase cost-effectiveness, integrate hospital data for test algorithms and strategies, more business management in addition to technical management, more interactions with physicians on test ordering and utilization, more effective needs assessment for our services, close relationship with near-patient testing services, maintain and increase scientific and technical capabilities, develop genetics testing, outreach orientation, be a leader in distribution of new scientific knowledge about laboratory testing, move out of the hospital, willingness to look at our competition, improved testing with higher information yield, eliminate tests with low information content, reflexive testing, develop new tests with higher information content, become a resource for development of clinical laboratory science.

Brainstorming is a useful technique in determining what we want or need to become.

It was decided that, at the end of the training program, a small team would be charged with developing a vision statement based on this information, with the suggestions of using an affinity diagram and other management planning tools such as a tree diagram. This did not prove to be an easy process. Gaining consensus on a laboratory vision was one of the most difficult tasks we undertook. Perhaps this is to be expected in any academic organization where many of the faculty and section directors have their own visions that have different degrees of alignment with the service, teaching, and research missions of the organization.

Managing TQM Momentum (Session 6)

In this training session, we reviewed the laboratory efforts to implement TQM, assessed that we had implemented many of the elements in steps 1 through 5 of the GOAL/QPC 10-step implementation plan, identified the next steps with an emphasis on understanding the faculty and section directors' roles in implementing TQM, used force-field analysis to identify the supporting (driving) and opposing factors that affect our progress, and discussed strategies for moving forward. We recognized it might be necessary to change some of the methods and approaches that had been developed in the early phases of implementation. We needed to integrate

We needed to integrate TQM into our regular work activities and make it a part of the way we did our work.

TQM into our regular work activities so that it was no longer considered as a separate activity, but was the way we did our work. This meant substantial changes in our organizational culture. We had the traditional academic laboratory structure by clinical discipline or section. The narrow section-oriented approach by the faculty and section directors promoted competition rather than teamwork. We needed a culture that allowed us to make changes both within and across sections, encouraged employee cooperation and participation across sections, and developed shared governance with empowerment of the employee closest to the daily work.

The brainstorming exercise identified the following driving forces: JCAHO's new quality standards, fulfillment of our laboratory mission, personal initiatives to improve service, competition driving improvement, and cost containment as a way of life. The restraining forces identified included the following: old habits; suboptimal empowerment of our staff; employee's lack of belief that their input is valued; lack of support from the hospital, medical school, and university; cost containment; need for education and training; other obligations of faculty and directors.

Of these restraining forces, one that was within our control was the need for training and education. Strategies that were identified for reducing this restraining force included reducing employee turnover, developing TQM self-study modules, functioning as role models for our staff, providing opportunities for continuing education, using the University of Wisconsin office of quality as a training resource, developing less complex processes, improving productivity to allow more time for training, making training an integral part of the process, and organizing hospital-wide training.

There was considered discussion and ideas about adapting the current TQM training for managers and supervisors. We established this opportunity as the next training priority. It was clear that the faculty and section directors felt the current training needed to become more "hands-on" if it was to be effective with managers and supervisors. They recommended a 2- to 3-day workshop format rather than the course's short periods of an hour and a half during a 10-week period. The need for practical examples relevant to laboratory medicine was emphasized, rather than the examples from other businesses that were included on the videotapes in the faculty and section directors training course.

Achieving Breakthrough Objectives Through Hoshin Planning (Session 7)

The GOAL/QPC model emphasizes three major systems for TQM: cross-functional management, daily management, and Hoshin planning. Most of our initial efforts supported daily management by means of project teams, the introduction of the seven basic tools, and efforts at continuous improvement and standardization. The next major system we needed to improve was strategic quality planning. GOAL/QPC's Hoshin planning approach emphasized organizational breakthrough, vertical teams and horizontal coordination, and the use of the seven management and planning tools.

"Hoshin Kanri" is a Japanese term that means "shining metal" or "pointing direction," such as from a compass. This is intended to point the organization in the right direction for its future growth and development. The American term that is used for this type of planning is "breakthrough" planning. Hoshin planning is directed by top management, but is accomplished by involving the whole organization in designing and implementing improvements in targeted areas. The key is to envision the future organization and then identify these most important strategic objectives for moving in that direction.

"Hoshin Kanri" means "shining metal" or "pointing direction."

GOAL/QPC describes the Hoshin planning process with the following steps: (1) establish organizational vision; (2) develop a 3- to 5-year plan; (3) develop annual objectives; (4) deployment by rolling down to departments to develop detailed plans; (5) implementation; (6) progress review; (7) annual review, with feedback to step 3, which then starts the yearly cycle again. The benefits of Hoshin planning include creation of a systematic process for yearly breakthrough planning, deployment of breakthrough objectives down the organization, improved communication through "catch-ball," periodic monitoring of the implementation, and annual adjustment and refocusing of the breakthrough objectives and strategies for implementation.

The planning process is supported with seven management and planning tools—the affinity diagram, interrelationship digraph, tree diagram, matrix diagram, prioritization matrices, process decision program chart, and activity network diagram—which are illustrated in Figure 2-6. We distributed a book, *The Memory Jogger Plus*,[7] that provided detailed procedures and examples of these management and planning tools. We also purchased the GOAL/QPC videotapes that demonstrate the use of these tools by a planning team. These tapes make it possible to provide instruction on the particular tool at the time when the tool is to be used by the team.

The planning process is supported with seven management and planning tools.

In our experience, the affinity diagram is particularly valuable because it provides a way to group and summarize items collected by brainstorming. We then often use a tree diagram to map out systematically the major categories of items and work toward finer details in case we missed anything in the brainstorming exercise. The matrix diagram has many uses in assessing the relationships among items, establishing responsibilities, and assigning tasks. The activity network diagram is a good tool for summarizing and describing a plan.

The affinity diagram is a particularly valuable tool.

Figure 2-6.
Seven management
and planning tools
(with permission from
GOAL/QPC, Methuen,
MA 01844).

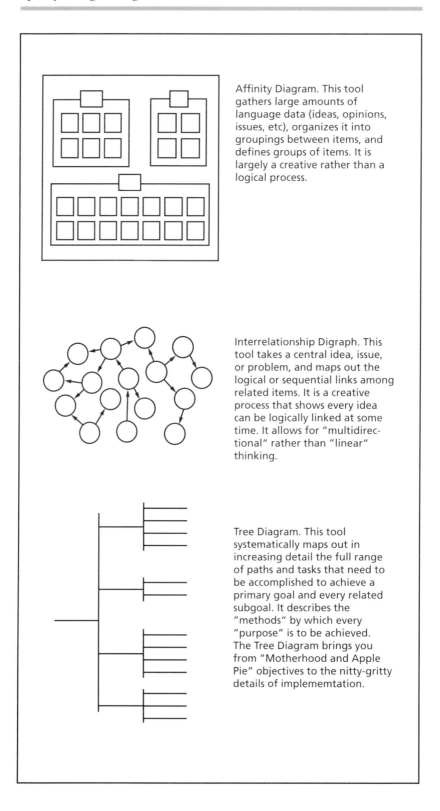

Affinity Diagram. This tool gathers large amounts of language data (ideas, opinions, issues, etc), organizes it into groupings between items, and defines groups of items. It is largely a creative rather than a logical process.

Interrelationship Digraph. This tool takes a central idea, issue, or problem, and maps out the logical or sequential links among related items. It is a creative process that shows every idea can be logically linked at some time. It allows for "multidirectional" rather than "linear" thinking.

Tree Diagram. This tool systematically maps out in increasing detail the full range of paths and tasks that need to be accomplished to achieve a primary goal and every related subgoal. It describes the "methods" by which every "purpose" is to be achieved. The Tree Diagram brings you from "Motherhood and Apple Pie" objectives to the nitty-gritty details of implememtation.

Figure 2-6, continued.

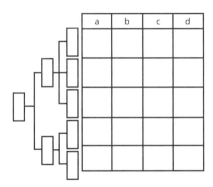

Matrix Diagram. This tool organizes large amounts of information such as characteristics, functions, and tasks into sets of items to be compared. By graphically showing the logical connecting point between any two or more items, a Matrix Diagram can expose relationships between items. Beyond the existence or absence of a relationship, it can also code each relationship to show its strength and the direction of influence.

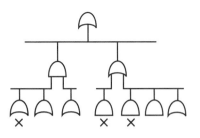

Prioritization Matrices. These tools prioritize tasks, issues, product/service characteristics, etc, based on known weighted criteria using a combination of Tree and Matrix Diagram techniques. Above all, they are tools for decision making.

Process Decision Program Chart. This method maps out conceivable events and contingencies that can occur in any implementation plan. It in turn identifies feasible countermeasures in response to these measures. This tool is used to plan each possible chain of events that need to occur when the problem or goal is an unfamiliar one.

Figure 2-6, continued.

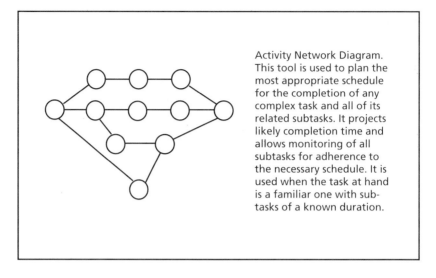

Activity Network Diagram. This tool is used to plan the most appropriate schedule for the completion of any complex task and all of its related subtasks. It projects likely completion time and allows monitoring of all subtasks for adherence to the necessary schedule. It is used when the task at hand is a familiar one with subtasks of a known duration.

Daily Management and Standardization (Session 8)

"Daily management" involves both teams and individuals.

In the GOAL/QPC model, "daily management" is the component for "unit optimization," which involves both teams and individuals in the continuous improvement of their work processes. Daily management is described as including an obsession with customers to understand process requirements, standardization of processes, training in tools for continuous improvement of processes, metrics for measuring process performance, and creation of high performance teams.

As applied in our laboratory, the team process was reasonably well developed but we lacked a formal mechanism for involving individuals in continuous improvement and supporting their efforts. Informally, many of our analysts contributed new ideas and improvements in the routine fulfillment of their responsibilities. The real issue was one of recognizing these efforts and stimulating ongoing and widespread contributions from individual employees.

The GOAL/QPC manual on daily management by Moran, Collett, and Cote[8] was provided to our faculty and section directors, along with some additional handouts that Collett provided during a subsequent visit to the campus. Collett described critical processes as "the important sets of procedures or patterns of tasks that determine success (customer satisfaction) for an organization or for an individual's job." She identified the following attributes of critical processes: they usually number 5 to 10; they are linked, both horizontally and vertically; they can be mapped or diagrammed; they can be measured; and they can be improved.

Daily management is perhaps most easily understood as the application of the principles and tools of TQM to one's own work processes. This may involve teams formed around the work processes of a group, as well as individuals focusing on processes that have a high level of individual ownership. Because both applications depend on an understanding of critical processes, most of this session reviewed and reinforced the concept of critical processes. Collett suggested that typical management of critical processes would include the communication process, barrier removal process, team participation and sponsor process, performance recognition and reward process, evaluation process, and training process. Specific laboratory examples were given based on a 1974 early paper on quality management from our laboratory: "Achieving quality is everyone's job."[9] These critical quality management processes included selecting personnel, planning/developing service processes, providing in-service training, delegating authority for service processes, and establishing a supportive culture, as outlined in more detail in Table 2-2.

The application of critical processes to the work of the faculty and section directors was illustrated·by the affinity diagram in Figure 2-7. This was based on the earlier brainstorming exercise in training session 3. The activities identified as critical for faculty and section directors were grouped into the following categories: plan laboratory operations, develop personnel resources, develop service processes, and provide patient care services. With this as a starting point, we developed the tree diagram in Figure 2-8 to review and expand the definition of critical processes. The "plan operations" category was expanded to include fiscal management, training, and long-range planning; "develop personnel" was expanded to include training and obtaining resources; "develop service processes" was expanded to include training, reporting functions, reducing complexity, evaluating utility, ordering, and communication with physicians to determine customer needs; "provide patient care services" was expanded to include monitors, consultation, interpretation, and guidance on test selection. New categories that were identified included "teaching/education," "quality assurance and monitoring," and "research."

A similar approach could be used to formulate critical processes for managers. In an initial brainstorming exercise, the following activities were identified: scheduling, standardization, troubleshooting, personal development, recruitment, production, manage the main event, quality assessment/quality control (QA/QC), motivation, communication, feedback, technical expertise, and continuing education. Time during this session did not permit further development, but the next steps would have included preparing an affinity diagram and then a tree diagram. In this way, critical processes could be defined for different levels of management in our laboratory.

Daily management is the application of the principles and tools of TQM to one's own work processes.

Table 2-2.

CRITICAL PROCESSES FOR MANAGING QUALITY.[9]

Selecting personnel
Assessing capabilities through teaching/training experiences
Communicating expectations to candidates

Planning/developing service processes
Defining quality requirements
Determining critical process characteristics
Deriving process specifications
Establishing method selection criteria
Establishing method evaluation protocols
Designing control procedures
Standardizing protocols for routine service

Providing in-service training
Assigning specific training responsibilities
Defining the training process
Preparing training materials
Providing systematic training experiences

Delegating authority for service processes
Establishing critical processes for each analyst
Supporting individual development
Recognizing individual contributions
Supporting work groups (natural teams)
Recognizing team contributions

Establishing a supporting culture
Providing continuing education and training
Delegating authority to individuals
Providing feedback on individual performance
Recognizing individual contributions

New Cross-Functional and Functional Teams (Session 9)

The terms "cross-functional" and "functional" take on different meanings depending on one's view of the organization. We consider laboratory project teams to be cross-functional when they have members who represent many different laboratory sections; however, the hospital would view such teams as functional if all the members were from the

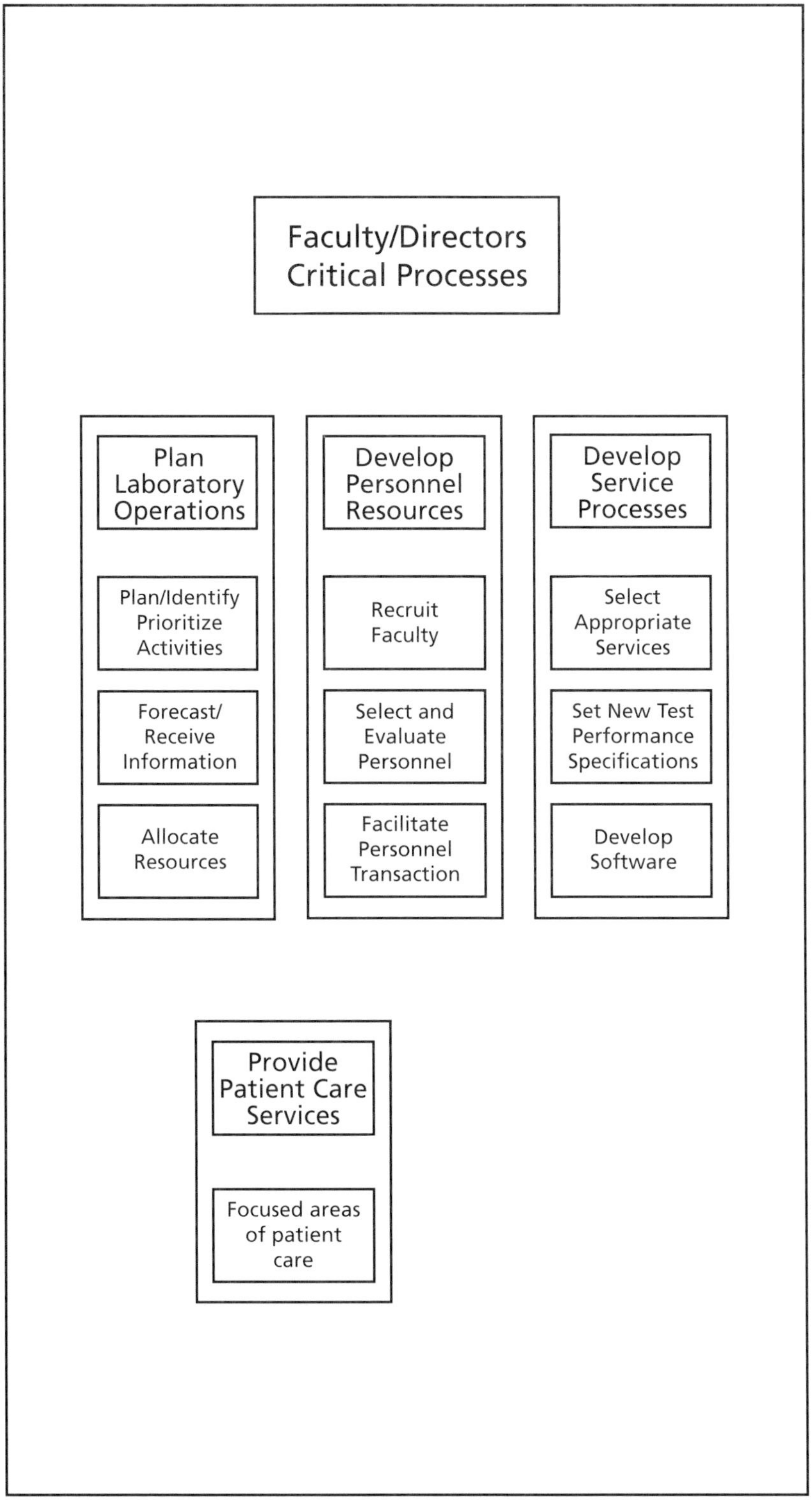

Figure 2-7.
Example "affinity diagram" of critical processes for faculty and directors.

Figure 2-8.
Example "tree dia-gram" of critical process for faculty and directors. CLS = clinical lab science; MT = med-ical technologist.

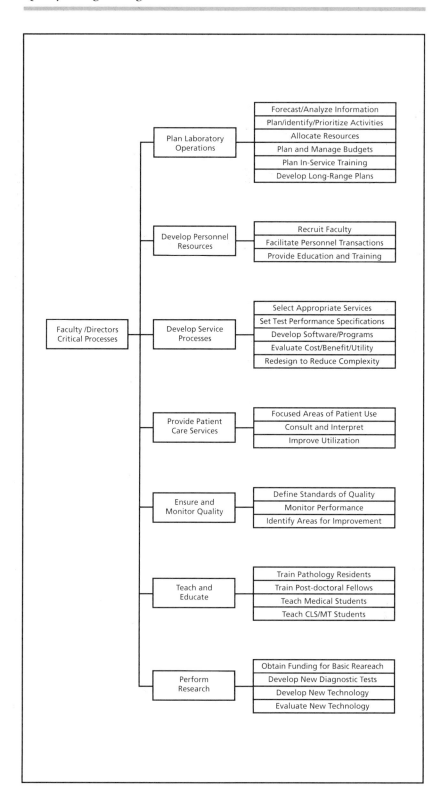

laboratory. In the context of our laboratory, functional teams are the section teams that are part of the daily management component of TQM.

Cross-functional teams are often organized to promote the organization's Hoshin or breakthrough objectives. For the six laboratory Hoshins that had been identified at the time, cross-functional teams were assessed to be useful for coordinating our efforts in the areas of (1) establishing molecular probe technology, (2) improving systems by reducing complexity and increasing automation, and (3) implementing the daily management component of TQM. There were existing faculty groups and academic mechanisms available for (4) improvement of educational programs. We made management assignments for (5) implementation of an effective outreach program. Finally, individual faculty responsibility was essential for (6) increasing research capacity.

A deployment matrix was developed to relate the interests of individual faculty and directors to the six Hoshins and to identify the appropriate team members. Technical interests and expertise identified the group responsible for establishing molecular probe technology. Many of these individuals had specific responsibilities for test menus that would profit from this technology; thus a natural, but informal, team already existed in this area. A somewhat different group was interested in improving systems by reducing complexity and increasing automation. This Hoshin eventually led to a series of teams and the reengineering effort in our laboratory.

To implement the daily management component of TQM, two cross-functional teams were needed. The existing QST was a cross-functional team with overall responsibility for supporting TQM implementation. Discussion of daily management identified some existing groups and committees that served the roles of functional teams in some areas. Differences between teams and committees were discussed, with the major distinctions being identified as the structured team problem-solving process and training in tools and techniques for quality improvement. A new cross-functional team for daily management was clearly needed to achieve breakthrough in this specific area. Because this involved activities within laboratory sections, we decided that the daily management team be developed as an outcome of our manager/supervisor training course.

Review TQM Progress and Revise Implementation Plan (Session 10)

This final session reviewed and summarized the status of our TQM implementation activities and identified three areas of focus for the next year: (1) daily management, (2) Hoshin or breakthrough planning, and (3) "save time" quality improvement projects. Our updated implementation plan was described by the activity network diagram shown in

Figure 2-9. Daily management would be launched following the next training program for managers and supervisors. They would be expected to establish a daily management project team to guide its implementation. Breakthrough planning would begin with a retreat for faculty, directors, and laboratory administrators. Quality improvement (QI) projects would continue under the guidance of the QST.

We began planning for GOAL/QPC training for managers and supervisors immediately. It was to be accomplished within the next 3 months. This training was condensed to $2^{1}/_{2}$ days and was presented twice to accommodate work schedules and to maintain smaller groups. Further training for all our staff was envisioned within the next year as an outcome of daily management and was to be accomplished before we launched our reengineering efforts. Our training staff ran full-day workshops several times to provide training for the 200 employees in our laboratory.

The laboratory director concluded the course with a quote from Deming: "Hard work and best efforts, put forth without guidance of profound knowledge, leads to ruin in the world that we are in today. There is no substitute for knowledge." After 10 sessions and about 15 to 20 hours of training and discussion, many of the faculty and section directors were still divided over their understanding of the full implications of TQM. Some were still fearful of the time and effort that would be required for further implementation and were hesitant to commit the resources of their sections to a more formal daily management program. Others believed that the team approach was essential to our future and that TQM was a management approach that needed to be pursued vigorously.

There is no substitute for knowledge.

LESSONS LEARNED

Our training efforts taught us the following:

Absolute necessity of providing training and education.

- We learned the absolute necessity of providing training and education about the overall plan, philosophy, tools, and techniques if we were to make major changes in our organization.

- The use of a nationally recognized program (GOAL/QPC) lent authenticity as well as structure to our efforts, reinforced our earlier experiences about quality management and the importance of the team process, and provided tangible examples to clarify points of instruction.

- Involving several of our own staff in the instruction spread the work around, brought their energies and interests into the process, and strengthened their commitment.

- The training sessions were well received by our staff, as evidenced by the remarkably few absences throughout the pro-

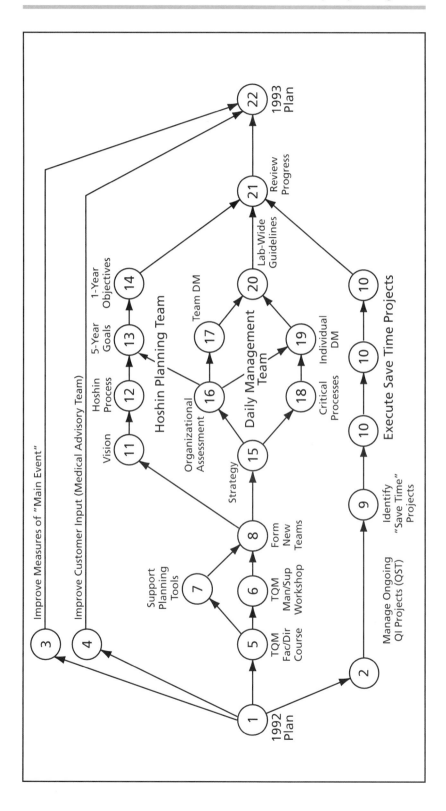

Figure 2-9.
Example "activity network diagram" of plan for implementing TQM. TQM = total quality management; DM = daily management; QI = quality improvement; QST = quality steering team; Fac = faculty; Dir = director; Man = manager; Sup = supervisor.

gram. Our employees at all levels responded to the program because it was rational, used the scientific method, provided workable tools and techniques, and empowered each staff member to evaluate and improve his or her role in the organization.

- Illustrative of our success was the formation of many informal work groups that improved their processes, such as the one used to evaluate instrumentation in hematology.

- The downside was the great time commitment by laboratory employees at all levels. It was sometimes difficult to maintain our workflow while asking employees to attend classes. Most of the extra reading was done on the employees' own time; however, the complaints about these requirements were few and each section willingly helped to provide time for its staff.

A surprising lesson for management was the comprehensive nature of TQM.

There was also a surprising lesson for management. We gained an added appreciation of the comprehensive nature of TQM and the GOAL/QPC approach. At times, we felt overwhelmed by the detailed requirements and the need to balance so many things at the same time. In fact, we did not have the resources to move in all directions at the same time. Thus, we were constantly making choices about which path to emphasize. One such example was our decision to complete the GOAL/QPC training and move to "daily management" before formally implementing "Hoshin planning." The choice was made because we believed we had articulated goals and that we needed to engage the bench worker as soon as possible.

Politics often presented obstacles.

We also learned the value of including representatives of hospital administration and recognized the potential usefulness of also including the department of pathology and laboratory medicine and the school of medicine in a more formal way. The politics and rapid changes occurring in the department and the medical school often presented obstacles that we could not overcome.

Nevertheless, we had moved forward and had set the stage for reengineering by developing a focus on processes, providing a team-oriented approach, and introducing the Hoshin idea of breakthrough planning.

REFERENCES

1. Total Quality Management Master Plan: An Implementation Strategy. GOAL/QPC research committee 1990 research report no. 90-12-02. GOAL/QPC, 13 Branch Street, Methuen, Mass 01844, 1990.

2. Westgard JO, Wiebe DA. Cholesterol operational process specifications for assuring the quality required by CLIA proficiency testing. *Clin Chem.* 1991;37:1938–1944.

3. Westgard JO, Hytoft Petersen P, Wiebe DA. Laboratory process specifications for assuring quality in the U.S. National Cholesterol Education Program (NCEP). *Clin Chem.* 1991:37:656–661.

4. Westgard JO. Charts of operational process specifications ("OPSpecs charts") for assessing the precision, accuracy, and quality control needed to satisfy proficiency testing criteria. *Clin Chem.* 1992;38:1226–1233.

5. Westgard JO. Analytical quality assurance through process planning and quality control. *Arch Pathol Lab Med.* 1992;116:765–769.

6. Westgard JO. A program for assessing statistical control procedures. *Med Lab Observ.* 1994;26(2): 55–60.

7. Brassard M. *The Memory Jogger Plus: Featuring the Seven Management and Planning Tools.* GOAL/QPC, 13 Branch Street, Methuen, Mass 01844.

8. Moran JW, Collett C, Cote C. *Daily Management: A System for Individual and Organizational Optimization.* Methuen, Mass, GOAL/QPC; 1991.

9. Westgard JO, Hunt MR. Achieving quality is everyone's job. *Laboratory Management.* 1974;20:595–602.

Planning for Strategic Breakthrough

CHAPTER 3

BACKGROUND

Although our program of total quality management (TQM) had brought significant improvements to the clinical laboratory, we eventually concluded that more fundamental changes were required to meet the challenges of the new health care environment.

In the first chapter of this book, we described the national and local health care conditions present in 1988 and 1989. In addition to these general statements, there were several more specific conditions that influenced our decision to move ahead with our reengineering efforts.

Madison is the capital of Wisconsin and sits in Dane County. Up to 70% of the county's population is served by one of four health maintenance organizations. The remaining 30% of the population is served by traditional fee-for-service medical care. In addition, several businesses had formed a health care alliance to seek lower rates for their 70,000 employees. Capitated care, ie, medical coverage for an annual fixed fee per enrollee, had begun to emerge as an important economic determinant for health care providers. Finally, there had been mergers and takeovers of hospitals and smaller health care units throughout the state. Health care providers were being pushed to become more cost-competitive and efficient.

From 1991 through 1992, the federal government had implemented the Clinical Laboratory Improvement Act of 1988 (CLIA-88).[1] The implementing regulations produced a great emotional and financial impact on laboratory practices. Although the regulations had relatively little effect on well-run, large laboratories such as ours, it demanded that all laboratories adhere to the same standards. This was difficult for some smaller laboratories and particularly many of the physicians' office laboratories (POLs). Consequently, CLIA-88 provided opportunities for larger laboratories to consult with smaller operations to meet the demands of the law in an economically viable manner.

Implementation of CLIA-88 required an increased administrative burden for all laboratories. Merger of laboratories would, at least in theory, reduce the overall administrative costs for the combined entities.

Fundamental changes were required to meet the challenges of the new health care environment.

Capitated care, ie, medical coverage for an annual fixed fee per enrollee, had begun to emerge.

The University of Wisconsin Hospital and Clinics (UWHC) Clinical Laboratory was a highly complex, sophisticated laboratory. Our university hospital physicians demanded that we offer state-of-the-art assays. We also performed many reference assays for the other laboratories in our community. We reasoned that we could improve our economic competitive position by increasing our role as a reference site for the three other HMO/hospital laboratories, the adjacent Veterans' Administration facility, and the many smaller laboratories in the area.

In addition to looking outward for new business, we felt that we needed to ensure that our internal functions were efficient. Changing the basic design of clinical laboratories is not a new idea. Howard Rawnsley, MD, developed a "core" facility for the Dartmouth-Hitchcock laboratory in the 1970s, and James Winkelman, MD, had partially achieved such for the Brigham Hospital Laboratory in the late 1980s. Commercial laboratories had developed along industrial principles rather than following traditional clinical or academic dogma. Indeed, our new laboratory director suggested that a core laboratory be developed at UWHC in 1988 but received vociferous objections from faculty and laboratory staff. The laboratory director discussed this dilemma with Dr Rawnsley, who strongly advised that the proposal be held in abeyance until there was more support, particularly from the supervisory staff.

We became aware of several important technological developments that might be applied to the clinical laboratory.

Meanwhile we and other laboratorians became aware of several important technological developments that might be applied to the clinical laboratory. These included optical scanning of labels (bar coding) and the general field of robotics. Of course, computer hardware and software continued to advance, particularly in memory storage and speed. Masahide Sasake, MD, PhD, of Kochi Medical School and the Japanese government worked together in a private-public partnership to develop a model automated/robotics laboratory.[2] North American laboratorians became aware of Dr Sasake's remarkable facility through visits and video tapes. In addition, several Japanese commercial outfits, particularly IDS and Hitachi, were beginning to produce off-the-shelf products for clinical use.[2]

In this country, James Boyd, MD, and Robin Felder, PhD at the University of Virginia Health Sciences Center developed a robotics blood gas facility.[2] This facility was to be used near the patient wards, with the apparatus activated by scanning an ATM-like card. In addition, the facility was connected to the main laboratory computer for quality control, release of data, recording, and billing purposes.

In addition to these technological advances, another major scientific advance was also taking place, the introduction of molecular biology into the clinical arena and specifically the clinical laboratory. The first wave of diagnostic molecular pathology allowed for the more accurate diagnosis of hematologic malignancies by determining which germline genes (B- or T-cell lymphocytes) were rearranged. It was apparent that this was only the tip of a huge iceberg and one that the university's department of pathology and laboratory medicine could not ignore.

Thus, the convergence of finances, politics, law, technology, and science provided the need for us to reexamine our assumptions and redefine the clinical laboratory.

PATHWAY TO THE CORE LABORATORY
Developing the Vision

Systems Analyses.—We approached two different sources for help in analyzing the work flow in the laboratory. The first was an industrial engineer, Jerry Sanders, PhD, in the School of Engineering at the University of Wisconsin.

After several discussions with Dr Sanders, we agreed to assign a team of industrial engineering students the task of examining the work flow in the clinical laboratory and making recommendations for improvements. This practical experience was to meet one element of their degree requirements.

We also sought help from industry. Several manufacturers in the United States were approached about developing automated systems in the clinical laboratory. We originally intended to include more than one firm to explore problems through planning, model building, and performing pilot projects; however, the need to share information was a major stumbling block and eventually only one company, Kodak, was willing to work in this more open configuration.

Kodak and the industrial engineering students developed somewhat different projects. Each group worked with us and cooperated with each other. Thus, several students, directed by Dr Sanders of the university's industrial engineering department, and Michael Spang (clinical products division) and Karen Leroy (management services division) from Kodak along with members of our staff began to formulate projects. Richard Coolen of Kodak provided support through the use of computer modeling.

Our goals were to improve the quality, safety, and efficiency of the clinical laboratory. A 9-month time-line was developed. Two separate reports were generated and each contributed to our understanding of the current laboratory work flow and its complexities.

The report by the Kodak-UWHC team set the agenda for most of the reengineering program. The team suggested the following as benchmarks for any changes:

* Decrease laboratory turnaround-time

* Decrease personnel time in processing samples

Convergence of finances, politics, law, technology, and science provided the need for us to reexamine our assumptions and redefine the clinical laboratory.

Our goals were to improve the quality, safety, and efficiency of the clinical laboratory.

- Reduce the number of times a sample is handled

- Increase the capacity to handle fluctuations in laboratory work flow

- Reduce laboratory errors

- Improve cost position of the laboratory.

The team segmented laboratory flow into seven discrete steps; however, the studies concentrated on three: (1) specimen acknowledgment (log in, label generation, sample receipt and tracking), (2) internal laboratory sample processing (laboratory information system, centrifugation, sample splitting, etc), and (3) analysis (performing the test).

Both computer and manually generated data were collected, compared, and analyzed. At the UWHC, most of the outpatient samples were collected and sorted in an outpatient laboratory facility located near the clinics and about a 5-minute walk from the main laboratories. The team studied this laboratory first, to gain experience with the process before investigating the larger and more complex central laboratory.

The outpatient laboratory included the main phlebotomy drawing and storage area, specimen receiving and entering, and chemistry and hematology analyzers (Figure 3-1). The work flow of the outpatient laboratory proved to be more complex than anticipated (Figure 3-2). Because we were also preparing to implement a bar coding program, the team was able to analyze laboratory processes before and after the bar coding program was implemented. The team found that bar coding reduced the throughput time by about 20%. Some of the gains were unanticipated, likely because of freed-up time being applied to other tasks and improved morale (Figure 3-3).

Before studying the central laboratory, a study plan was suggested, discussed, and established by members from Kodak, UWHC, and industrial engineering. The laboratory was segmented into phlebotomy, specimen control, chemistry, and hematology for this study. The study team toured each section, and a series of combined workshops were held with two representatives from each site. During the first 2-hour meeting, the enlarged team brainstormed all its activities. These were then put on post-it notes and placed in sequence. Each section explained its flow to the other groups. Each individual was then revisited for clarification and expansion of the work flow. Later in the week, the whole group met again to review and revise the flowcharts. A final draft of the study plan was prepared by the team.

Findings.—As expected, turnaround-time was correlated with work load and these fluctuations led to creative uses of personnel scheduling. Thus, at the major peak of activity, between 6 AM and 9 AM, the

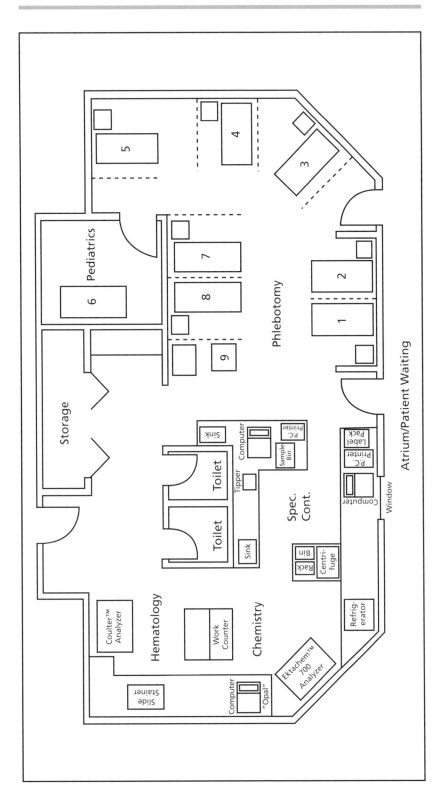

Figure 3-1.
The layout of the outpatient laboratory showing the phlebotomy and laboratory areas. Spec. Cont. = specimen control.

Figure 3-2.
This flowchart of the activities in the outpatient laboratory showing the numerous steps involved in collecting and testing patient specimens and the interconnection between the steps. Note: dashed lines represent time data collected.

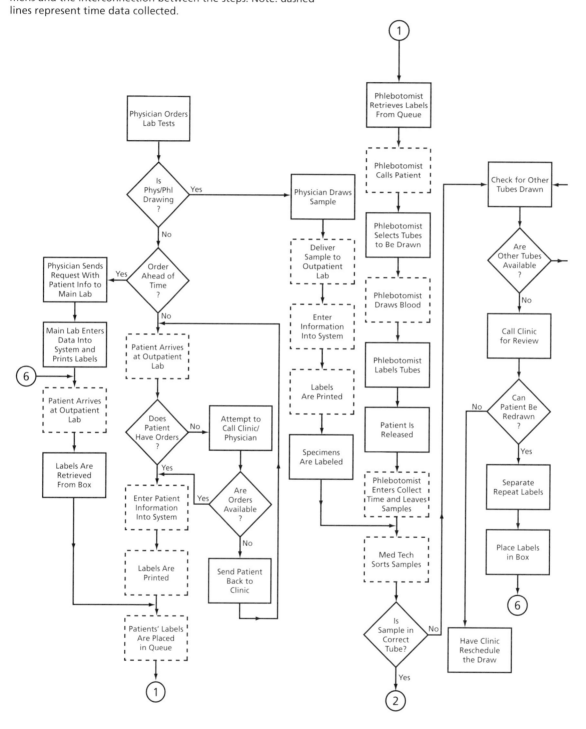

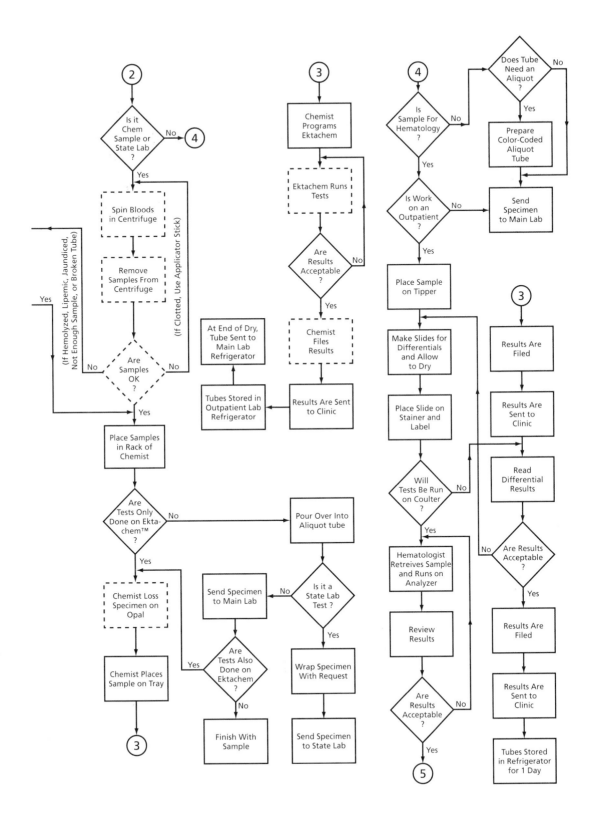

Figure 3-3.
A bar chart showing the results of studies before and after the introduction of bar-code labels for specimen tubes in the outpatient laboratory.

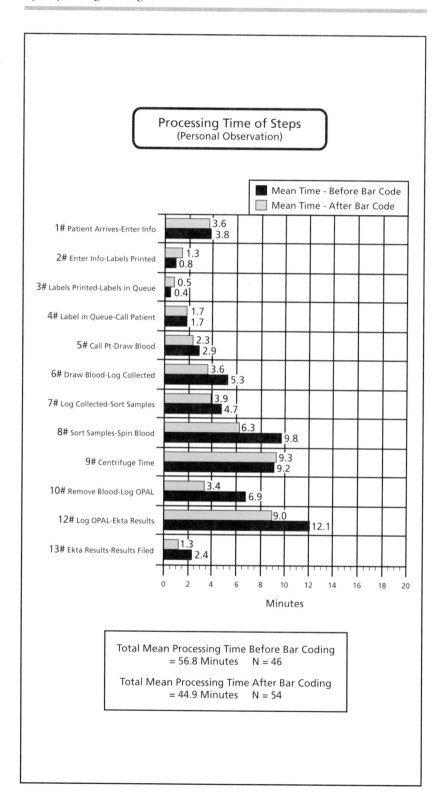

Processing Time of Steps
(Personal Observation)

■ Mean Time - Before Bar Code
□ Mean Time - After Bar Code

1# Patient Arrives-Enter Info — 3.6 / 3.8

2# Enter Info-Labels Printed — 1.3 / 0.8

3# Labels Printed-Labels in Queue — 0.5 / 0.4

4# Label in Queue-Call Patient — 1.7 / 1.7

5# Call Pt-Draw Blood — 2.3 / 2.9

6# Draw Blood-Log Collected — 3.6 / 5.3

7# Log Collected-Sort Samples — 3.9 / 4.7

8# Sort Samples-Spin Blood — 6.3 / 9.8

9# Centrifuge Time — 9.3 / 9.2

10# Remove Blood-Log OPAL — 3.4 / 6.9

12# Log OPAL-Ekta Results — 9.0 / 12.1

13# Ekta Results-Results Filed — 1.3 / 2.4

Minutes
0   2   4   6   8   10   12   14   16   18   20

Total Mean Processing Time Before Bar Coding
= 56.8 Minutes   N = 46

Total Mean Processing Time After Bar Coding
= 44.9 Minutes   N = 54

turnaround-time was slower than that for the rest of the day. A less intense peak of activity was associated with an intermediate turnaround-time.

In addition to work volume, we compiled a laundry list of contributors to variation in time for processing and performing samples. These included differences in order forms and specimen containers, illegible handwriting, mislabeled tubes, insufficient quantities of blood, and drawing in the wrong tube. The team also identified transport of samples to the laboratory as a significant deterrent to improving turnaround-time. Samples were picked up on the wards on a scheduled basis and transported by hand to the clinical laboratories, which had no input into the scheduling of the transporters.

In addition, there were two within-laboratory processes that were identified as major obstacles to improving turnaround-time: preparing aliquots and centrifuging samples. The team further concluded that the work area layout was not conducive for rapid responses.

Concurrently, a separate laboratory team was investigating ways of alleviating the interruptions caused by the 350 phone calls per day the laboratory received or the need to print results on an "as needed" basis.

The team also discovered that there was no set policy on the acceptability of samples, ie, hemolysis, jaundice, and lipidemia; that the laboratory had no system to track samples throughout the process; and that there was confusing redundancy in the chemistry section with as many as four methods for a single analyte and accompanying methods of control, logs, and paperwork.

Recommendations.—The team presented its recommendations in the form of a three-phase plan. The recommendations generated from these studies provided the conceptual basis for our future actions as shown below.

Recommendations generated from these studies provided the conceptual basis for our future actions.

- Phase I: Standardization of the Inputs and Outputs of the Specimen Control Section.—The goal of this phase was to standardize specimen collection, laboratory procedures, and laboratory equipment. Specific recommendations included (a) reducing the number of blood collection tubes and the number of subsequent sample aliquots, (b) extending the bar coding program not only throughout the laboratory but also onto patient sites, (c) improving sample transport to and within the laboratory, (d) simplifying the priority system, (e) moving ahead with the development of a phone center, and (f) consolidating the analyzers in the clinical chemistry section. The team believed full implementation of the bar coding program and integration of it into the laboratory information system would improve sample tracking and reduce paper records.

- Phase II: Grouping of Analyzers and Equipment by Throughput and Technical Capabilities.—The goals of this phase were to group instrumentation by level of automation rather than clinical discipline and to transfer as many measurements as possible to the more automated, random access machines. In addition, the team suggested that more automated specimen processing systems be investigated.

- Phase III: Automated Specimen Processing and Laboratory Transport Devices.—The goals of this phase were to automate specimen processing and transport fully within the laboratory so that work would be prioritized and specimens routed, tracked, stored, and retrieved.

Developing a Consensus

The laboratory had defined some of its major objectives. In retrospect, this was the easiest part of the process. We needed to fill in the details of the plan and gain the support of hospital administration and our laboratory staff and colleagues. We moved from our roles as engineers and scientists to become salesmen. Several activities occurred concurrently.

We moved from our roles as engineers and scientists to become salesmen.

Retreat.—After many discussions with the section directors and managerial staff as well as hospital administration, we recognized the need to bring these entities together at one time and in one place to "gain consensus on organizational changes for meeting future laboratory needs." Thus, on March 12, 1993, we held a one-half day, off-campus retreat. Participants included the section directors, some key laboratory managers, and the senior hospital administrator assigned to help manage the laboratory.

There were four major objectives of the retreat: (1) understand the financial imperatives and hospital expectations for laboratory service; (2) identify possible future organizational modes; (3) clarify issues that affect laboratory operation; and 4) determine future organizational changes.

The format included reports and materials distributed before the retreat, presentations by administrators and section directors to reveal their perspectives, a question and reply session to clarify issues and reports, and a discussion period to develop priorities for the next steps.

A large amount of materials were provided to each participant so that all would have the requisite background information for informed discussion, dialogue, and decision making. These materials are described below in some detail.

1. Franklin Elevitch's "The Fourth Dimension. Management of the Postmodern Clinical Laboratory" describes the four complexities of contemporary laboratories, legal, technical, medical, and now managerial.[3]

2. The medical center had formed a managed care task force that made recommendations to the medical school faculty. It suggested that the center move into managed care as rapidly as possible. The task force emphasized the needs to develop quality standards for service, an integrated information system, and effective mechanisms for cost management with future investments.

3. The laboratory director and several retreat participants described the various relationships among and between hospitals, laboratories, and medical schools in this country.

4. The laboratory space committee reviewed space needs and availability. It suggested that the laboratory immediately begin eliminating duplicate instrumentation.

5. The laboratory personnel team reported on its survey of personnel needs at peak and off-peak times in the laboratory and supported the concept of cross coverage.

6. The director of data processing updated the status of the development of a new laboratory information system. He emphasized that the hospital's administration would not support the continuing development of another generation of the current system. Some options were suggested and discussed. It was determined that the existing system probably could not be supported beyond 1997.

7. The laboratory phone team presented a plan to establish a phone center without increased personnel.

8. The laboratory outreach planning committee updated our current efforts in point-of-care and reference testing.

9. The daily process management team outlined the three tracks of its pilot project.

10. We reviewed the background and rationale for the laboratory automation workshop to be held in June 1993 in Madison.

11. The laboratory's goals and objectives for 1993 through 1994 given to hospital administration in January was distributed.

The hospital's associate superintendent provided his perspective and emphasized the medical center's changing financial picture. He urged the laboratory to look at several items carefully: labor costs including less expensive employees, cross training, and automation; organizational structure, particularly reducing the management layers; and management of support services and fixed costs.

The laboratory director emphasized the complexities of the laboratory's relationships with the hospital and medical school and the need for increased flexibility. He predicted the need for a more flexible, rapidly responsive, competitive organization with more reference testing and a greater consultative role.

A round-robin discussion followed in which all participants contributed their comments and recommendations. After all contributions were heard, we asked if there was agreement that reorganization was necessary. Such a consensus was obtained with the proviso that reorganization would contribute to our future viability. The laboratory director then condensed the ideas into five discrete goals: (1) reduce operating costs; (2) enhance "outreach"; (3) maintain and enhance professional careers; (4) encourage research, development, and technology transfer; and (5) increase clinical consultation.

From this time forward, the laboratory leadership reiterated, extended, and clarified the goals generated from this retreat. The retreat participants had asked that a team be named to continue the change process. Thus, the laboratory director named a team to review laboratory processes and make concrete and temporal recommendations for change.

The laboratory director named a team to review laboratory processes and make concrete and temporal recommendations for change.

The Clinical Laboratory Process Review Team.—The "process review team" consisted of the directors of quality assurance and data processing sections and a technologist whom we had trained in the use of computer simulation. The team was charged with reviewing the tests, methods, instruments, personnel use, space, and work flow patterns within the clinical laboratories. The team was to report on the current activities of each section and to recommend changes based on anticipated savings in positions, space, equipment, supplies, and time. The team was to seek breakthrough opportunities rather than incremental improvements. The method employed involved meeting with each section director or manager to get an overview and his or her responses to a series of questions designed to aid in understanding the section's operations. One person from each section was assigned to work with the team as it gathered more detailed information on tests, methods, instruments, personnel, work flow, and space. The team spent considerable time observing the operations within each section. After data gathering, the team wrote a preliminary summary of activities that was presented to each section for review, comments, clarification, and correction. The corrected sum-

The team was to report on the current activities of each section and to recommend changes based on anticipated savings in positions, space, equipment, supplies, and time. The team was to seek breakthrough opportunities rather than incremental improvements.

maries along with recommendations constituted the final report, which was prepared and presented to the laboratory director about mid-September of 1993. The chronology of activities generated from the process review team is shown in Figure 3-4.

The report from the process review team consisted of several pieces: reiteration of methods, general findings, specific recommendations, and supporting documentation. The most important finding of the process review team was confirmation of our belief that the people working at the bench were functioning efficiently. Our efforts in TQM and daily process management continued to improve the effectiveness of the laboratory and its personnel. Thus, any major improvements were not likely to occur under the current systems. The team identified several constraints on further improvements, which included demands for patient care, limitations of analytical methods, regulatory requirements, fixed costs, capital equipment costs, space, demands for university programs, and maintenance of a highly trained workforce. The team further focused on three areas for consideration: (1) streamlining the analytical processes in the laboratory, (2) reducing noncost effective laboratory testing, and (3) increasing the efficiency of the teaching efforts. The laboratory had the most control over the first of these areas and the team suggested that tests be done by the most cost-effective technology that meets medical decision requirements, backup and alternative procedures be reduced, low volume tests be sent out unless the volume can be increased via reference testing, and outdated tests be eliminated.

The process review team gave 21 discrete recommendations to reorganize the laboratory to achieve real change (Table 3-1), the cornerstone being development of a high volume, rapid turnaround-time core laboratory.

The team presented and discussed the report with the laboratory director and his advisory group. After study of the report and discussions with other section directors and management consultants, the director elected to remove the organizational structure components of the report before passing it on to the rest of the laboratory staff. This was done to keep the focus on the process of developing a core laboratory rather than prematurely placing a management structure on an incompletely defined entity.

Catchball.—Catch-ball is a TQM term used to describe the process by which ideas are "thrown" to a person or group, which then reviews and possibly adjusts the thought before throwing it back to the original pitcher. We used this process for dialogue and consensus among the laboratory section directors, managers, staff, and administrative structure.

The most important finding of the process review team was confirmation of our belief that the people working at the bench were functioning efficiently.

Any major improvements were not likely to occur under the current systems.

The cornerstone to real change was the development of a high volume, rapid turnaround-time core laboratory.

Figure 3-4.
A time line showing the relationship among the various phases of the reengineering project.

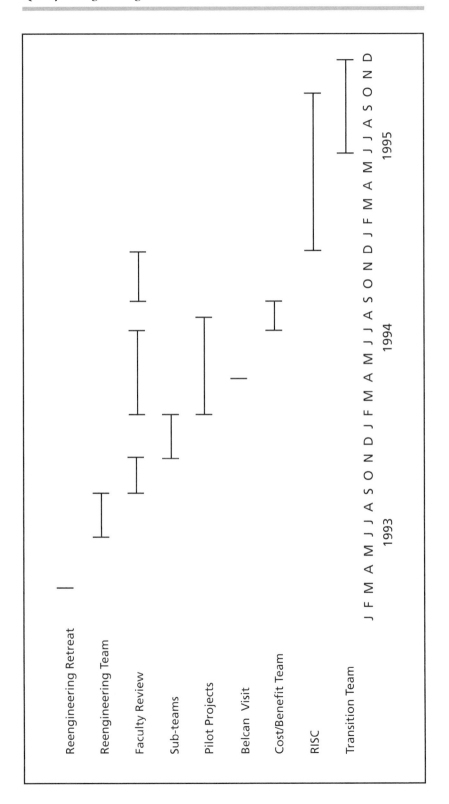

RECOMMENDATIONS OF THE LABORATORY REENGINEERING TEAM

Table 3-1.

I. Reorganize the laboratory into four management areas:

   A. Microbiology, histocompatibility, and transfusion service

   B. Four heavily instrumented sections:

   Core laboratory, batch laboratory, SSI (setup, storage, and information), and separations

   C. Labor intensive testing:

   special chemistry, special hematology, phlebotomy, immunology, and reference testing

   D. Support services:

   Data Processing, Quality Assurance, and Administrative Support

II. Create an Instrumented Laboratory Committee (ILC) that would manage the core laboratory, the batch laboratory, the SSI, and separations.

III. Create a Manual Methods Committee (MMC) that would manage special chemistry, special hematology, phlebotomy, immunology, and reference testing.

IV. Create a Support Services Committee (SSC) that would manage data processing, quality assurance, and administrative support.

V. Install mechanical conveyors to bring work to the core laboratory in 2 to 3 minutes from selected points in the hospital.

VI. End laboratory work in the outpatient laboratory and remodel the space as office and work space for phlebotomy.

VII. Move molecular diagnostics, heavy metals, and low volume testing in chemistry such as fecal fats and electrophoresis to another site.

VIII. Create a high volume core laboratory whose function would be to turn out the maximum number of test results in the least amount of time.

IX. Adopt a point-of-care testing policy to minimize stat requests from inpatient units.

X. Place all the batch analyzers together into one laboratory section called the batch laboratory.

XI. Create a setup, storage, and information (SSI) section around the nucleus of the current specimen control.

XII. Create a new separations section around the nucleus of the current toxicology section.

XIII. Create a new immunology section by merging the nonautomated work in current immunology section with the flow cytometry section.

XIV. Create special chemistry around the nucleus of the current endocrinology laboratory, including the gyn/endo laboratory.

XV. Create a special hematology section that does manual differentials, slide review of various types, bone marrows, and special coagulation studies.

XVI. Revamp the services offered at University Station.

XVII. Consolidate the management of all quality control, workload recording,

Table 3-1, continued.

proficiency testing, quality assurance activity, validation, calibration procedures, and statistical analysis into the quality assurance section.

XVIII. Reevaluate quality requirements for patient care.

XIX. Reduce the number of different sized vacutainers and develop precise standards for all specimen containers in use.

XX. Improve data processing for histocompatibility, bone marrow, and microbiology.

XXI. Review the laboratory organization on a biannual basis.

The one area over which there was no disagreement was the need to develop a high volume, highly efficient core laboratory.

In mid–October 1993, the process review team report was presented to the laboratory section directors who were asked to respond. A dialogue using memoranda and e-mail ensued during the next 2 weeks. There were 24 discrete comments/concerns made by the section directors. The laboratory director collated these into four larger categories: vision, structure, information, and implementation. The one area over which there was no disagreement was the need to develop a high volume, highly efficient core laboratory. All comments were distributed to the section directors before their meeting at the end of October.

At this session, after a brief review of the process team plan, ie, the need for change induced by finances, the opportunities for change afforded by technology, and the goal of providing more opportunity for faculty development, we focused on the practical aspects of developing a core laboratory. The round-robin discussion technique was used at first to allow each member to make one or two points that he or she felt were critical. We then entered a period of general discussion with many "what if" questions raised and answered. While we all agreed on the need to do something, we were unable to come to a consensus before the meeting adjourned; however, we did agree to meet again for that purpose as soon as possible (10 days later). At the second meeting, a consensus was finally reached as each alternative was explored and found less attractive than the process team proposal. Two specific actions were agreed on: (1) distribution and discussion of the report with the laboratory managers and then the rest of the staff and (2) formation of five teams to define the core laboratory. The report was distributed with a cover letter providing some background. The laboratory director held two meetings with managers and three with the rest of the staff. In addition, each laboratory section discussed the plan at one or more meetings. In this way, the laboratory section directors were seen as supportive of the plan and integral to the future of the laboratory.

Detailing the Core Laboratory.—In mid-November 1993, five teams were charged with detailing and defining the core laboratory, which included the "Central Automated Routine and Emergency Laboratory" (CAREL), the "Automated Batch Analyzer Laboratory" (ABAL), and the "Setup, Information, and Storage Laboratory" (SISL).

Team one was to select instrumentation; team two to develop staffing; team three to select specimen transport, processing, and storage equipment; team four to simulate the work flow in the core laboratory to aid the other teams; and team five to develop quality management for the laboratory. By March 1994, all teams had completed their reports.

Instrumentation.—There were three laboratory section directors/faculty, one of whom was appointed team leader, and three senior medical technologists on this team. The team was to propose instrumentation and its configuration for the core laboratory. It was to consider maximizing random-access instruments while maintaining precision and accuracy; guaranteeing backup for critical assays; maximizing batch analyses; minimizing the number of different technologies, particularly for the same analyte; maximizing the use of our current equipment; and using the most cost-effective methods including reagents, training, space, and quality control. After reviewing the current work flow and volumes, the team presented three possible configurations; all included current automated chemistry, hematology, endocrinology, coagulation, and microbiology instruments arranged in plasma, whole blood, and serum lines of operation. The third configuration sought to incorporate potential new instruments (Figure 3-5).

Staffing.—There were two laboratory section directors/faculty, three senior medical technologists, and a hospital administrator (human resources) on this team. One of the faculty members was appointed team leader. The team was charged with defining tasks to be done in the different parts of the core laboratory and then developing a supervisory model. The team's third task was to estimate training needs as personnel jobs are changed. The staffing team was asked to work in concert with both the instrumentation and modeling teams. This team never met its charges. Its only contribution was to encourage the retraining of current laboratory personnel rather than hire new personnel for open positions—a policy already adopted. This failure was due chiefly to the choice of team leader, the only faculty member who did not endorse the development of the core laboratory. The failure was costly because it required development of another team to estimate cost savings.

Transport.—The transport team consisted of five senior medical technologists, including those involved in phlebotomy and specimen recording, tracking, etc. In addition, there was one representative from

Figure 3-5.
The initial sketch of the core laboratory concept showing the reorganization of the work and the use of a conveyor to move specimens. Chem Anal = chemical analyzer; Endo Drug = endocrinology and drug testing; SSI = setup, storage, and information.

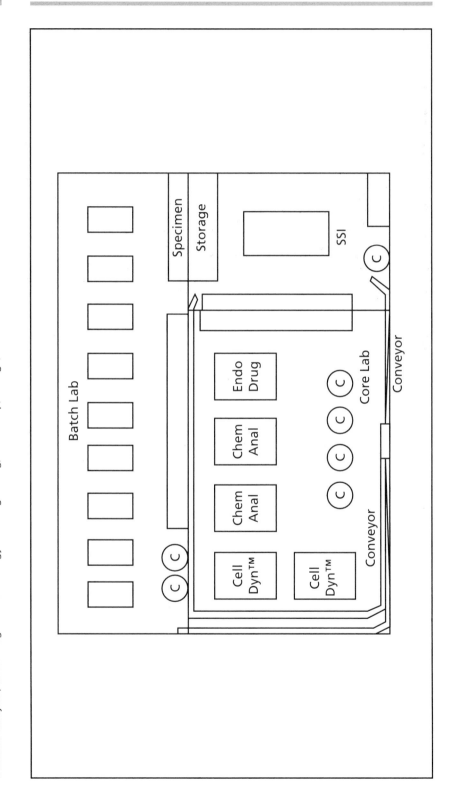

hospital administration. This team was to identify vendors for and information about processing equipment, ie, sorting, centrifuging, etc; moving samples to and between laboratory analytical stations; and storing and retrieving patient samples. In each case, the team identified the vendors and compared availability of equipment, the completeness of the system, cost, volume/hour, integration of instrumentation, places of current use, maintenance, downtime, construction costs to install, quality assurance monitors, restrictions, and likely impact on personnel. In addition, it recommended a new layout for the core laboratory.

Work Flow.—The work flow team was composed of one faculty member and three medical technologists, including one trained in the use of computer simulation. The team was charged with obtaining specimen arrival, processing, and analytical timing data to allow the development of simulation models. This team was to work closely with all other teams as they proceeded in their tasks. There was no formal report from this team.

Quality.—The composition of this team included one faculty member or section director, four senior medical technologists, and a member of the laboratory data processing staff. The charge to this team was to determine the need for a uniform and systematic approach for managing quality of all testing in the core laboratory and to identify the required support services. The team developed an affinity diagram listing the quality management support services (Figure 3-6). It then constructed a matrix that listed which persons had the primary, secondary, or "needed-to-know" for each of the services. From the matrix, a "quality" job description was developed for each personnel level, from the bench technologist to the director of the laboratory medicine section.

More Catch-ball/Pilot Studies.—The faculty/section directors and managers/supervisors were provided with these reports and commented on them. In February 1994, the laboratory initiated several pilot studies to test some of our earlier assumptions. One study compared the efficacy of near-site testing for blood gases with similar testing done in the main laboratory using pneumatic tubes. It revealed no difference in turn-around-times, provided the tubes were dedicated to the laboratory and convenient for dropoff. A second study compared sample preparation, including centrifugation, "up front" with preparation at the site of the instrumentation. There was a significant savings in turnaround-time if samples were processed at the site of the instrument. The third pilot study attempted to reduce the number of medical technologists needed on a third shift with increased cross-training. This study demonstrated that a 20% personnel saving could be effected, ie, 1.4 of 7.0 full-time employees (FTE). We began to integrate instrumentation previously used in other sites into the main laboratory. This action was neutral, ie, there were no notable changes in service or personnel needs.

It revealed no difference in turnaround-times, provided the tubes were dedicated to the laboratory and convenient for dropoff.

There was a significant savings in turnaround-time if samples were processed at the site of the instrument.

Figure 3-6.
Quality management support services. PT = proficiency testing; CE = continuing education; DLM = division of laboratory medicine; MT = medical technologist, MLT = medical laboratory technician; QC = quality control; NBS = National Bureau of Standards; CAP = College of American Pathologists.

Quality Management Support Services

Maintaining Regulation/Accreditation

- standardizing procedure manuals
- maintain Proficiency Testing program
- standardize how we handle PT specimens
- coordinating accreditation/inspection process
- uniform policies and procedures for monitoring quality
- define, develop, and implement quality assessment monitors
- investigate occurrence screen and correction report complaints

Standardizing Test I/O

- standard request process
- minimize type/size of specimen tubes
- Minimize number of specimen tubes drawn per patient
- specifications for specimen labeling
- standardization of specimen labeling
- standardize communication of problem samples to next processing area
- explore minimal path of specimen
- standardization of specimen policies and procedures
- uniform reporting policies
- standardization of specimen transportation

Maintaining Workforce

Staff Development

- cross-training or standardizing training
- coordinate CE activities throughout DLM
- standardize new employee orientation
- investigate cross-training between areas
- continue to address recruitment/retention issues
- maintain work environment which supports quality work
- standardization of safety policies and procedures

Staffing Issues

- organizing work responsibilities
- decision on centralization of responsibilities (needs to be broken down)
- determine levels of staff (MT, MLT, quality)
- staffing for computer support
- establish means of handling phone calls

Figure 3-6, continued.

Maintaining Total Quality Control

- maintain statistical QC system
- standardize QC assessments
- standardize out of control situations
- standardize patient QC activities
- provide training in computerized QC programs
- establish uniform preparation of QC materials (preparation, check-out, ranges)
- standardize QC and coordinate QC schedules
- standardizing function checks, (ie, temps, thermometer checks, pipettes)
- standardize type and use of pipettes and automatic diluting devices
- standardize and coordinate instrument maintenance schedules
- determine frequency of QC of back-up methods
- uniform calibration verification
- maintaining alternate calibration and method verification materials (NBS, CAP)
- minimize number of different calibrators, verifiers, and control materials
- standardize linearity verification

Selecting and Verifying Methods

- define Quality Requirements
- selection of instruments
- define criteria for placing tests in defined areas
- assess feasibility of moving tests
- optimize number of systems doing same test
- define extent of verification needed
- verifying/evaluating methods/instrument
- establishing procedures for validating changes to existing methods/systems
- reference value studies

Managing Materials

- define responsibility for maintaining inventory of consumables
- standardization of consumables
- combine ordering of QC products and bid process
- standardize procurement procedures
- standardize reagent labeling policies and procedures
- standardizing workload recording

Information Processing

- develop specifications for computer support (hardware, staff needs)
- manual vs. online operation
- implement "bidirectional" communication
- automatic review of test results
- change and standardize computer information (worksheets, logs, loadlists, on-line operation)
- design requisition order logic
- coordinate maintenance/ update of computer systems
- maintaining availability of information systems
- specimen tracking system includes time, location, condition
- patient QC checks
- statistical QC systems
- Proficiency Testing database
- database query system
- automatic integration of separate reports (bone marrow, State Lab, reference labs, others)
- statistical routines
- resource scheduling system (maintenance personnel, QC)
- test order monitors
- monitor patient treatment factors (drug administration, cross-reactivity, heparin, arterial lines)

The laboratory section directors and staff were ready to move ahead to begin an ambitious reengineering program; however, hospital administration and the acting chair of the department of pathology and laboratory required a more detailed estimate of costs and savings. Thus, in July 1994, we charged a team to prepare a cost/benefit analysis of a core laboratory. This report was completed in mid-September 1994.

Cost/Benefit Analysis.— The director of data processing led this team, which also included two supervisors, two experienced "bench" technologists, and a technologist trained in computer simulation. Members were chosen because of their past experience with teams, detailed knowledge of one or more sections of the laboratory, and demonstrated willingness to accept change. All the laboratory section directors and faculty served as consultants and the laboratory director was an ex-officio team member. An interim report in August 1993 summarized the activities of each section relative to a core laboratory, reiterated the services to be delivered by the core laboratory, and started to list specifically the types of instruments required in the core laboratory. These were the criteria recommended for inclusion into the core laboratory:

1. High volume

2. Testing available at all times

3. Automated, "routine" assays

4. STAT testing

5. Barcoded primary sample

6. On-line (with computer) instrumentation

7. Minimal sample preparation

8. Similar technology for many assays

9. Easy maintenance of operator skills

Those test attributes that would be relatively detrimental to inclusion in a core laboratory included:

1. Dependent on a "special" technique

2. Manual

3. Requires microscopy

4. Low volume

5. Requires batch testing

6. Requires interpretations or reviews

7. Specialized customer-oriented activities (sendouts)

The core laboratory menu also included assays that although of low volume, could be performed rapidly and with minimal expertise.

The final report gave 37 specific recommendations, each with costs and projected savings. An estimate of the effects of these changes on all laboratory sections and an estimate of the personnel required to staff the core laboratory (83.5 FTE vs existing number for the same tasks, 89.9) were also included. The team recommended that we consider developing the core laboratory in two phases: (1) start-up in the main laboratory and (2) integration of the outpatient laboratory into the central facility. Overall, there was an estimated reduction of the entire laboratory staff by 7% to 8% with both phases fully implemented. There was an estimated annual supply saving of 3% in the laboratory's total supply costs. There were one-time savings in replacement of three major instruments of at least $150,000. Finally, there were associated costs of $1,040,000 with the three largest items being laboratory space renovation, and inter- and intra-laboratory transport/processing systems.

There was an estimated reduction of the entire laboratory staff by 7% to 8% with both phases fully implemented.

This report was presented to and discussed by the faculty/section directors who supported the findings with some reservations. The laboratory director, with the laboratory advisory group, developed an implementation action plan based on the accumulated data.

Action Plan.— The laboratory director presented the cost/benefit findings to hospital administration to obtain its endorsement. In addition to the financial implications, the report emphasized the need to pursue study of (1) other laboratory areas (ie, microbiology, transfusion medicine, molecular diagnostics, and histocompatibility) and (2) transport systems within the hospital. We estimated net savings for phase I (excluding outpatient laboratory) of $98,000 for year 1 (assuming implementation over a 6-month period) and $776,000 for year 2. The estimated savings for phase II (including outpatient laboratory) were $420,000 in the first year and $410,000 for year 2. We estimated yearly savings of $1,186,000 when both phases were fully implemented.

We estimated net savings for phase I (excluding outpatient laboratory) of $98,000 for year 1.

We estimated yearly savings of $1,186,000 when both phases were fully implemented.

The next step in the action plan was to present the program to the laboratory managers and then the rest of the staff. Recall that these groups, particularly the managers, had multiple opportunities to comment on the change process. This was to be done as soon as hospital administration gave its support.

The third step of the action plan was to name a reengineering implementation steering committee (RISC). This was to be a joint effort by the laboratory and hospital administration.

The final component of the action plan was a reminder to continue parallel pathways in working with hospital, university, and State of Wisconsin personnel offices and the unions.

Hospital administration endorsed the reengineering program in early November 1994.

Pursuing the Action Plan.—Hospital administration endorsed the reengineering program in early November 1994. The laboratory section directors drafted and sent a letter to the laboratory managers (appendix) to provide the justification for a core laboratory and to present the financial assessment made by the cost-benefits team. The laboratory director, laboratory manager, and at least one section director then met with the managers on two occasions to present the plan and answer concerns and questions. There was guarded support.

This was followed by meetings of the laboratory director with each section. Ten meeting times were posted to allow staff to attend any one of the scheduled sessions. The laboratory director emphasized 10 key elements of the reengineering plan—

1. The laboratory sections most effected were chemistry, special chemistry, toxicology, hematopathology, microbiology, immunology, and specimen control.

2. There would be two receiving areas, one for inpatient samples and one for other samples (outpatient and research).

3. Samples would flow along two main lines, one for serum and one for whole blood (blood gases and hematology).

4. Most centrifugation and sample preparation would be done at the site of the instrument.

5. We would develop an internal transport system.

6. We would increase the use of bar coding.

7. There would be a cadre of core laboratory technologists who would be cross-trained to perform multiple functions under the supervision of a core laboratory manager.

8. Further specifics would be developed by an implementation team.

9. We aimed to initiate several items in this fiscal year including some renovations, cross-training, and some integration of services. We expected further implementation in the next fiscal year with completion of phase I from 1996 to 1997 and phase II from 1997 to 1998.

10. We expected to avoid layoffs unless the hospital had increased and unexpected financial difficulties. Downsizing would be accomplished by attrition and training our existing personnel in new skills. We expected that some of the savings would be reinvested in the laboratory, particularly in research and devel-

opment, to allow the hospital to remain competitive with other academic institutions.

The reengineering steering committee members were named by the laboratory director and senior hospital administrator, both of whom served on the committee. In addition, the head of hospital human resources, the laboratory senior manager, and four section directors were also asked to serve. The laboratory director was the chair and an administration employee, an experienced team facilitator, served in that capacity. A group dealing with the chemistry core efforts was also named to report to RISC.

REFERENCES

1. US Dept of Health and Human Services. Medicare, Medicaid, and CLIA Programs; regulations implementing the Clinical Laboratory Improvement Amendments of 1988 (CLIA). Final rule. *Federal Register.* February 28, 1992;57:7002–7186.

2. Eggert A, Ross P, Sobocinski P, Tomar R, Westgard J, eds. *Proceedings of the Clinical Laboratory Automation Workshop.* Madison, Wis: University Industrial Research; 1993.

3. Elevitch F. The Fourth Dimension. Management of the postmodern clinical laboratory. *Clinics in Laboratory Medicine.* 1992;12: 849–859.

Parallel Pathways

Expanding Influence

INTRODUCTION

This section might be subtitled "Meantime, back at the ranch . . . ." The path to reengineering for us was not a singular or linear one. Frequently we followed several paths, with some running parallel and some crossing at various points. We needed to learn more about the status of laboratory automation, pay increasing attention to internal and external outreach activities, solicit and engage our customers concerning their views about and needs from the laboratory, and work with employee unions as we moved toward change. In addition, we sought to obtain an external review about our plans.

THE CLINICAL LABORATORY AUTOMATION WORKSHOP— JUNE 1993

We organized an international workshop (*The Clinical Laboratory Automation Workshop,* Madison, Wis, June 6–8, 1993) to learn what was available or would soon be available internationally for laboratory automation. We also hoped to gain hospital administration support for restructuring the laboratory by exposing administrators to the advances being made in clinical laboratory automation. We hoped that the hospital administrators would appreciate the improvements in patient services as well as cost-effectiveness through the further implementation of automation. The workshop was sponsored by the University of Wisconsin Hospital and Clinics (UWHC), the University-Industry Research Program, and the College of American Pathologists (CAP), and it was held on the campus of the University of Wisconsin. The goals of the conference were to review the current status of clinical laboratory automation and to move toward the formation of a consortium to advance such systems. The program was developed by the laboratory medicine faculty with Philip Sobocinski (University-Industry Research Program). Representatives from academia, industry, and government contributed to the workshop. After opening remarks by representatives of the

We organized an international workshop to learn what was available or would soon be available internationally for laboratory automation.

We hoped that the hospital administrators would appreciate the improvements in patient services as well as cost-effectiveness through the further implementation of automation.

Table 4-1.

ESTIMATES OF LABORATORY ACTIVITIES

1989
- $80 billion (~13% of total health care costs)
- 50% hospital laboratories
- 25% physician office laboratories
- 25% other

1990
- 8.8 billion laboratory tests done in US
  HMO budget (Washington, DC)
- $35/enrollee/year for laboratory tests

three sponsoring organizations, the workshop was segmented into five data-presenting sessions followed by a wrap-up. The deans of the medical and graduate schools gave presentations at informal dinner meetings.

The first session provided background material (general session). Russell Tomar, MD, reviewed the history of clinical laboratories and provided some financial and organizational information (Table 4-1 and Figure 4-1). Mr Paul Mountain, vice president of science and technology, MDS Laboratories, summarized the initiatives in clinical analysis in Japan, particularly those of Dr Masahide Sasaki of Kochi Medical School. He also described the efforts of IDS, which had been in business for about 11 years and had about 30 applications available for clinical laboratories. William Godolphin, MD, professor of pathology, University of British Columbia, described programs in Italy, Switzerland, Scotland, France, Austria, and Germany. He also directed our attention to ISO-9000, an effort by the European community to develop standards in many areas including instrumentation. Neil Duffie, PhD, mechanical engineer and director of the Wisconsin Center for Space Automation and Robotics (WSCAR), then described future technological opportunities with the use of robotics and micromotors. Figure 4-2 shows an example of one analysis system in use by the United States space program. The final background element was provided by Philip Sobocinski on behalf of Gary Kramer, MD, National Institute of Standards and Technology (NIST). Mr Sobocinski described the Consortium on Automated Analytical Laboratory Systems (CAALS) outlined in Tables 4-2 and 4-3.

The workshop's second session focused on systems analysis and particularly aids to planning. James Westgard, PhD, from the University of

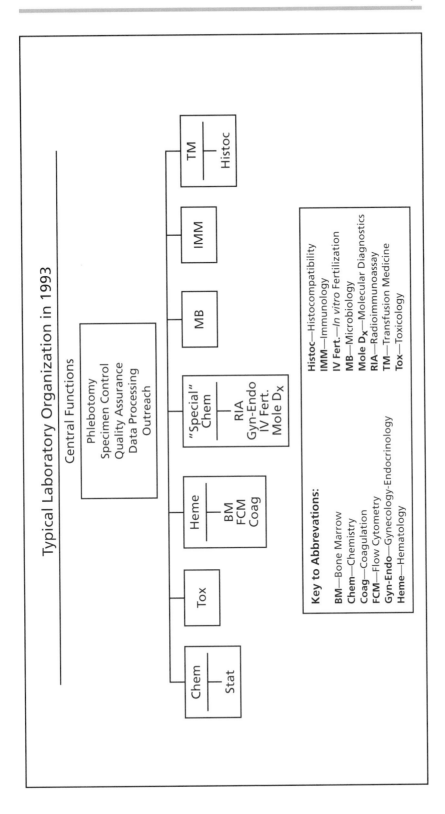

Figure 4-1.
Organization of a typical laboratory in the early 1990s. Note the emphasis on boxes or silos without many interlaboratory interactions. (With permission of Dr Russell Tomar, University of Wisconsin.)

Figure 4-2.
Organization of an
advanced spaced
robotics laboratory as
developed by the
Wisconsin Center for
Space Automation and
Robotics. (With permis-
sion of Dr Neil Duffie,
Wisconsin Center for
Space Automation and
Robotics.)

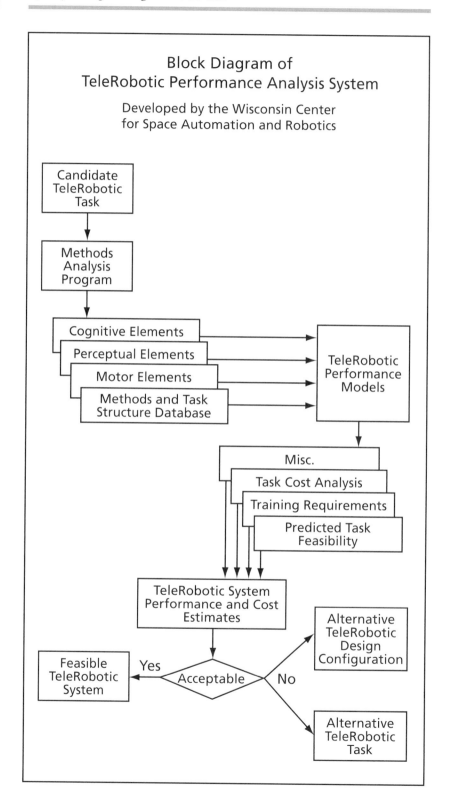

Block Diagram of
TeleRobotic Performance Analysis System

Developed by the Wisconsin Center
for Space Automation and Robotics

Candidate
TeleRobotic
Task

Methods
Analysis
Program

Cognitive Elements

Perceptual Elements

Motor Elements

Methods and Task
Structure Database

TeleRobotic
Performance
Models

Misc.

Task Cost Analysis

Training Requirements

Predicted Task
Feasibility

TeleRobotic System
Performance and Cost
Estimates

Feasible
TeleRobotic
System

Yes

Acceptable

No

Alternative
TeleRobotic
Design
Configuration

Alternative
TeleRobotic
Task

CAALS Research Objectives

- Develop the concept of modular analytical instruments as building blocks for automated analysis systems
- Promulgate standard specifications for automation and remote control of laboratory instruments and for connecting instruments to supervisory computer systems
- Automate common chemical laboratory procedures
- Create standard models for modular automated analytical instrumentation and for automated analysis systems
- Build quality assurance into the automated systems

Table 4-2. CAALS research objectives. (With permission of M. R. Rubin, National Institute of Standards and Technology.)

Current CAALS Research Topics

Modularity
- Concept of instruments as modules in analytical systems
- Specifications for interfaces between instruments and controllers
- Communications protocols and profiles
- Requirements for measurement system-information system interactions
- Sample management and tracking

Inorganic Applications
- Automated sample preparation
- Microwave-assisted dissolutions
- Flow injection sample processing
- ICP analyses

Organic Applications
- Automated sample preparation
- Supercritical fluid extraction of solids
- Automated fractionation of extracts
- Chromatographic analyses

Table 4-3. Current CAALS research topics. (With permission of M. R. Rubin, National Institute of Standards and Technology.)

Figure 4-3.
Line diagram indicating the factors to be considered for clinical quality planning. (With permission of Dr James Westgard, University of Wisconsin.)

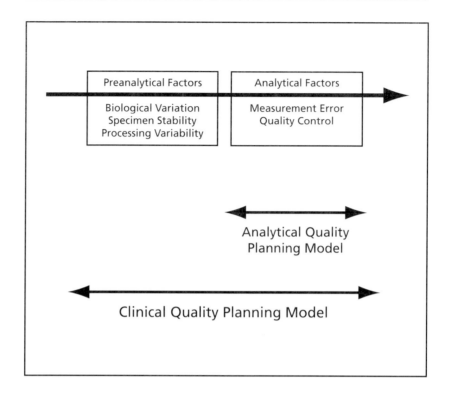

The ideal system would be the most automated, least costly, most flexible, most redundant, least spacious, least complex, and have the lowest maintenance with the easiest repair.

Wisconsin provided insights into quality planning models for the laboratory testing process, which are shown in Figure 4-3. Arthur Eggert, PhD, described the use of model simulation through computer programs such as that offered by ProModel (San Antonio, Tex). Dr Godolphin continued by sharing his experience in the use of simulations. Kevin Bennet from the Mayo Clinic revealed his organization's approach to automation and use of simulation. He concluded that the ideal system would be the most automated, least costly, most flexible, most redundant, least spacious, least complex, and have the lowest maintenance with the easiest repair. The system also would be nonproprietary.

Sample handling was the topic of the third workshop session. Denis Ferkany, president, Biomedical Devices Company, described the Automatic Aliquot System (Pontiac, Mich) (Table 4-4) that was developed by his company for SmithKline Beecham. Larry Maguire, MD, from Medical Robotics outlined his company's efforts to automate centrifugation and aliquoting. The manager of research and development of the C. S. Draper Laboratory, Edward Bernardon, demonstrated sophisticated use of robotics and other automated instruments in a class I clean-

FEATURES OF THE MODEL AAS AUTOMATED ALIQUOT SYSTEM BY BDC

Table 4-4.

- Closed tube specimen splitting protects laboratory personnel from serum exposure
- Automatically prints and applies test specific bar coded labels to aliquot tubes
- Processes 300 primary sample tubes per hour at an average of 2 aliquots per tube
- Aliquots variable test specific specimen volumes based on LIS data
- Multiple aliquot tube styles may be used with each primary specimen
- LIS interactive with remote requisition file database information
- Inverted primary tube process design allows for maximum specimen access
- Rack style sample management system ensures primary and aliquot tube split and match integrity
- Disposable CapTap™ device absolutely eliminates carryover concerns

Biomedical Devices Company patent 5,151,184 and patents pending.

room environment. George Nelms, vice president of engineering of AutoMed, Inc, talked about the development of his company's automated handling system (Arden Hills, Minn) (Figure 4-4).

There were three presentations in the fourth workshop session on automated analysis. The first was by James Boyd, MD, director of laboratory computing, University of Virginia Health Sciences Center. Dr Boyd emphasized four requirements of intelligent robotic systems: (1) sensors that might be present on robotic "hands"; (2) interfaces between robots, instruments, computers, and human users; (3) mobility to transport samples to instruments and results to customers; and (4) perhaps communications between instruments, robotics, conveyers, etc. Kenneth Whisler, PhD, director of laboratory information systems at Rush-Presbyterian-St Luke's Medical Center in Chicago, outlined that institution's program. The last speaker in this session was Rodney Markin, MD, from the department of pathology and microbiology, University of Nebraska Medical Center. The University of Nebraska Medical Center has developed a prototype laboratory automation platform that contains both chemistry and hematology analyzers using the paradigm of random-access specimen processing.

The fifth workshop meeting focused on systems integration. Mr Mountain and Stephen Middleton discussed the approach of MDS

Figure 4-4.
The automated handling system from AutoMed, as described by George Nelms. (With permission of G. F. Auchineck, AutoMed, Inc.)

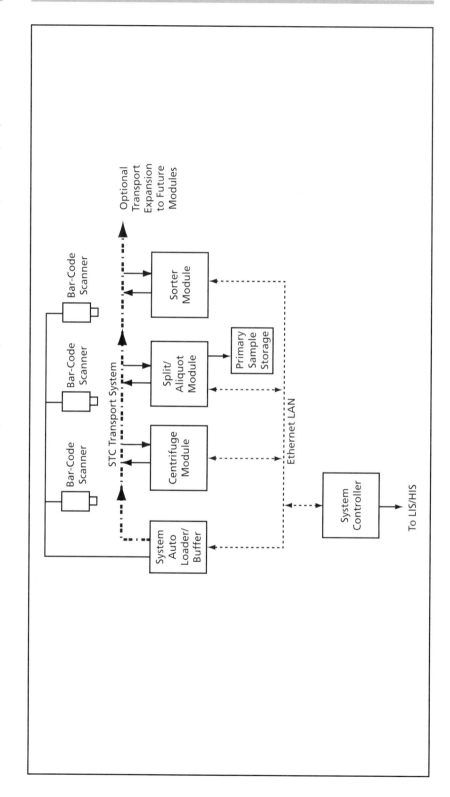

Table 4-5.

PURPOSES FOR A CONSORTIUM, AS SUGGESTED BY WORKSHOP PARTICIPANTS

1. Develop and recommend standards.
2. Identify problem areas.
3. Identify funding to address problems.
4. Share jointly acquired data.
5. Serve as a clearinghouse for information.
6. Gather resources.
7. Overall, move the field.

Laboratories, Toronto, to restructuring. They discussed four guiding company principles: (1) provide premier service; (2) improve quality and safety; (3) enable value contributions; and (4) service through automation, not to automation. Lowell Tilzer, associate medical director of the Community Blood Center of Greater Kansas City, Missouri, provided data for the value of thoughtful full implementation of bar coding, computerization, and instrumentation.

During the dinner before the final workshop day, questionnaires were distributed, described, clarified, and briefly discussed. These were collected and tallied the next day before the wrap-up session, which focused on requirements for advancing the field of laboratory automation. There were 32 responses to the questionnaire. Twenty-two of the participants supported some form of an industry/government/academia consortium to promote automation. All respondents were willing to participate in such a group if it were formed. Purposes for a consortium were developed by the audience and are provided in Table 4-5. Fourteen people volunteered to serve on the consortium steering team.

The Clinical Automation Workshop brought together many of the leaders in laboratory automation for presentations, discussions, and networking. It provided us with a realistic view of the "state-of-the-art" and confirmed our own opinions of the shape of things to come. Hearing the same theme from external experts helped convince hospital administration and the UWHC Clinical Laboratory section directors of the desirability, if not necessity, of restructuring. A subgroup of the participants later met in New Orleans with the support of the Becton-Dickinson Company and the American Association for Clinical Chemistry to develop a program for advancing clinical automation.

The participants supported some form of an industry/government/academia consortium to promote automation.

OUTREACH

There were three prongs to our outreach program: (1) oversight of point-of-care (POC) testing, (2) increasing our reference work, and (3) developing our own satellite laboratories. These approaches would take advantage of our experience and knowledge about laboratories, ie, legal, clinical, managerial, etc, and add value to the medical center by increasing revenues and competently supervising necessary services. Our first outreach position was filled by an employee who also served as supervisor of phlebotomy services, ie, it was a redefined position rather than a new one. Later, we added a second position as we increased the scope of our outreach. Still later, we separated phlebotomy from outreach because of the latter's continued development and the increased legal complexities imposed by the Clinical Laboratory Improvement Act of 1988 (CLIA-88).

Point-of-Care (POC)

CLIA-88 placed all laboratories performing assays for clinical use under federal regulation and standards. Thus, all laboratories, including those performing only a few tests, were required to obtain federal registration and accreditation. These rules conflicted with the increasing trend of testing closer to the patient rather than in a central laboratory. The trend was fueled by improving technology and the overlapping financial interests of manufacturers and health care providers. Manufacturers were interested in selling their new instruments, and providers could charge and collect laboratory fees instead of passing them on to a central laboratory.

POC or nearsite testing raised several important issues for medical centers. First, the quality (accuracy and precision) of the nearsite instruments was uneven.

POC or nearsite testing raised several important issues for medical centers. First, the quality (accuracy and precision) of the nearsite instruments was uneven, with many being clearly inferior to central laboratory testing equipment. However, even when the instrument itself performed well, a lack of experience, training, or interest by the operator led to inferior results. Second, results were often not posted on the patient's chart in a way that would allow other providers to have access to the information or they were not recorded in the official record of the patient, which at times led to redundant test ordering and presented other regulatory and legal issues. Finally, medical centers are frequently dependent on the revenues generated by a central laboratory. The total costs of nearsite testing might be the same or only somewhat greater than doing the same assays in the central laboratory; however, charges for performing these assays may not be recovered because of apathy, a lack of appropriate systems, or billing errors by the clinical department in the nearsite testing unit. Thus hospital revenues may be significantly reduced.

Hospitals operate under a self-regulatory body, the Joint Commission on Accreditation of Healthcare Organizations (JCAHO), which states that all laboratories within a hospital are the responsibility of the hospital and the laboratory director. Although this regulation is often ignored, CLIA-88 forced a new look and a change in behavior at the UWHC.

Federal regulations to implement CLIA-88 were not released until 1990/1991. During this period, we proposed that all laboratories at UWHC come under the oversight of a POC committee whose authority was based on a POC policy approved by hospital administration and the medical board. We were aware that other institutions were pursuing this same strategy.

Our concept was that the laboratory use its expertise to select instruments, train local operators, provide preventive maintenance, supervise proficiency testing, and oversee local operator skills. The central laboratory would provide the guidance for inspection and accreditation and ensure that all regulatory and legal issues were engaged. All data would appear on the patient chart with the appropriate site of performance provided. Appropriate charges would be developed and revenues equitably distributed.

Our concept was that the laboratory use its expertise to select instruments, train local operators, provide preventive maintenance, supervise proficiency testing, and oversee local operator skills.

Pediatric Intensive Care Laboratory.— We had an opportunity to test this approach before the final draft of the POC policy when the pediatric intensive care unit (PICU) requested that respiratory therapy be allowed to do blood gases. After discussions with the director of the PICU and review of several drafts, the following "experiment" was established:

- PICU was to identify space for a "stat" PICU laboratory.

- Respiratory therapy technicians would be available to perform assays 24 hours/day, 365 days/year.

- Laboratory medicine would select instruments in conjunction with PICU staff. These would be purchased through the laboratory's budget.

- Laboratory medicine would maintain the instruments, including preventive maintenance and troubleshooting as needed.

- Laboratory medicine would institute and maintain quality control and quality assurance. It would develop procedure manuals and methods for record-keeping.

- Laboratory medicine would organize and monitor proficiency testing programs.

- Laboratory medicine would train and accredit instrument operators.

- PICU and laboratory medicine would develop a method for billing and ensure that billing is performed.

- PICU with laboratory medicine would develop methods to restrict instrument access only to accredited operators.

- Laboratory medicine would be responsible for licensure and accreditation.

A cost analysis was performed and shared with hospital administration who agreed to a 6- to 12-month pilot program that would measure turnaround-times, proficiency testing results, and provider satisfaction. The extra time commitment by respiratory therapy was included in its annual report and budget preparations.

One of the laboratory technologists in the outreach section carefully trained, monitored, and eventually accredited 24 respiratory therapists to perform blood gases in the PICU laboratory. Results were included in the patient's laboratory reports and chart and appropriate billings were completed. Other than the cost of two new instruments in the PICU laboratory, there was no extra cost to the hospital. Turnaround-time improved and provider satisfaction greatly improved. PICU clinicians who had chronically complained about the tardiness of the laboratory's response, now became great supporters of this and other laboratory programs.

We compared turn-around-time in the PICU with turnaround-time for the same tests from the emergency department after a pneumatic tube was in place between the ER and the laboratory. Although there was no statistical difference between the times, the PICU staff remained more satisfied with its service.

As a follow-up to the PICU pilot, we compared turnaround-time in the PICU with turnaround-time for the same tests from the emergency department after a pneumatic tube was in place between the ER and the laboratory. Although there was no statistical difference between the times, the PICU staff remained more satisfied with its service.

The PICU laboratory had an impact on the central laboratory by requiring less personnel in the blood gas laboratory. It probably also extended the life span of the central laboratory's instruments. These savings are difficult to measure because there were other changes occurring simultaneously.

Point-of-Care Policy.—A POC Policy was adopted by the hospital medical board in May 1993. We had worked with a senior hospital administrator and the associate dean for clinical affairs, first determining the need and then writing, passing, and implementing the policy. The policy placed all hospital laboratory testing under the authority of the central laboratory. A procedure for obtaining authorization for noncentral-laboratory testing and an evaluation and implementation committee were established. The director of laboratory medicine was chair of this committee. The other members included the associate dean for clinical affairs, a senior hospital administrator, the medical technologist outreach supervisor, a representative of the hospital quality assurance department, and at least one practicing physician.

The medical board later approved another policy that affected near-site testing, ie, all instruments to be used for patient testing must be reviewed and approved by the laboratory or Point-of-Care Committee (POCC). This discouraged salesmen from selling directly to clinicians without appropriate review of quality, costs, regulatory requirements, and institutional policies.

Point-of-Care Committee.—The POCC was convened in August 1993. With the leadership of the associate dean and hospital administration, all clinical units were surveyed to determine the extent of testing not being done in the central laboratory. This survey took the political clout of the associate dean as well as the support of the chairs of the clinical departments and the medical board. The POCC was then charged with determining the level of testing and compliance with federal and other regulations. Thus each of the 20 to 30 sites were categorized as meeting or not meeting CLIA regulations and whether the site was performing wavered, moderate, or high complexity testing.

This survey took the political clout of the associate dean as well as the support of the chairs of the clinical departments and the medical board.

Nursing.—We had discussions with the nursing department to bring its extensive testing (urinalysis, glucometers, stool hematests, etc) into regulatory compliance. By July 1993, the laboratory and nursing departments had agreed to a plan that fell under the aegis of the POCC and the license of the central laboratory. Nursing and the laboratory staff developed a plan of training and oversight, in full compliance with CLIA-88, for approximately 1000 nurses. This was accomplished a few months after the decision to implement was made.

Nursing and the laboratory staff developed a plan of training and oversight, in full compliance with CLIA-88, for approximately 1000 nurses.

Other Hospital Units.— We have already discussed the PICU and the work with respiratory therapy. Similar operative agreements and working arrangements were developed with several other units including (1) dietary, which had been testing for cholesterol within the hospital but also at local malls and health fairs; (2) the gastroenterology clinic for "CLO" testing for *Helicobacter pylori*—the causative agent of gastroduodenal ulcers; and (3) the diabetes clinic for blood glucose and urine testing.

Nonhospital Units.—The clinical laboratory already had a separate license for one offsite laboratory that supported a UWHC specialty clinic called University Station Clinic. This laboratory included chemistry and hematology analyzers, computers, microscopy, phlebotomy, and three employees.

On August 1, 1994, after considerable negotiation, the laboratory at University Health Services, ie, the clinic charged with ministering to the University of Wisconsin student body, was brought under the licensure and direction of the UWHC Clinical Laboratory. This was done by a contract between the hospital and University Health Services and was the first time the clinical laboratory had been "allowed" to negotiate a contract with an external party. The University Health Services laboratory was placed under the purview of the POCC. The POCC and subsequently the University Health Services laboratory were reviewed by the hospital's quality evaluation and review committee (QERC). QERC in turn reported to the University of Wisconsin hospital medical board.

Inspection and Accreditation.—From 1991 through 1992, the clinical laboratory had been inspected and accredited, along with the rest of the hospital, by the JCAHO, a "private" organization whose regulations and rulings had financial and operative consequences to hospitals virtually equivalent to law. Alternatively, laboratories could choose to be inspected and accredited by the College of American Pathologists (CAP). Because its criteria were considered more stringent, most university hospital laboratories opted to come under CAP's mantle, which was accepted by JCAHO.

From 1991 through 1992, the clinical laboratory at the UWHC was inspected and accredited by CAP; however, JCAHO still inspected some parts of the main laboratory that it considered part of the professional component of the hospital. With the development of nearsite testing and new licenses, we needed to decide if we should place the POC laboratories under CAP or JCAHO regulatory requirements. We chose JCAHO because of the tardiness by CAP in adjusting its rules to make them applicable and palatable for nearsite testing. Some of the CAP general requirements for these smaller laboratories were onerous in scope and detail. Thus, the laboratories under the central laboratory license were CAP-accredited and all others were JCAHO-accredited.

The POC laboratories were inspected by JCAHO in the fall of 1994 and no serious deficiencies were found. A few lesser infractions were cited and addressed. The next inspection in the spring of 1996 found even fewer problems with none major.

POCC Cost Center.—Hospital administration agreed to develop a separate cost center accounting number and fund for POC testing. Thus, these laboratories' costs and revenues could be more readily tracked by the POCC and the hospital.

Provider Performed Microscopy.—As part of the CLIA-88 regulations, the Health Care Finance Administration (HCFA) added a new category of licensure, ie, physician (later provider) performed microscopy or PPM. Procedures requiring the use of the microscope were included. If one became licensed for these procedures, the licensee, also known as the director, could oversee other testing. Later, other groups, ie, nurse practitioners, physician assistants, etc, were also given authority to perform microscopy under the supervision of a physician. POCC developed a plan to bring these elements into compliance with federal

With the development of nearsite testing and new licenses, we needed to decide if we should place the POC laboratories under CAP or JCAHO regulatory requirements.

regulation. We first surveyed the medical center to determine the extent of compliance with federal regulation in testing. While several areas were in compliance, about 15 sites were either out of compliance or needed further clarification. One-by-one, each of the violations was addressed over a 3-month period until all units came into compliance. In addition, a discussion series was planned to review the regulatory requirements and responsibilities of the section directors of the POC laboratories.

About 15 sites were either out of compliance or needed further clarification.

Report to Quality Evaluation and Review Committee.—The POCC reported to the hospital's medical board through the quality evaluation and review committee.

Reducing the Price of Failure.— The licensures of the nearsite laboratories fell into three categories: (1) under the license and director of the central laboratory and historically administered and operated by the central laboratory; (2) under the license and director of the central laboratory but historically operated by another unit; and (3) under a separate license and director, not from the central laboratory.

Although we had no concerns about inspection and accreditation failures, we recognized that failures by those units covered by the central laboratory license and director were potentially the most troublesome because of the negative impact it would have on the central laboratory and hospital-wide services. Thus, we initiated a strategy to develop a second license and director under which all the laboratories in the second category and some of those in the first would be covered. By the spring of 1995, these laboratories were identified and placed under the license of the associate director of the clinical laboratory. Thus, a proficiency test failure by laboratories covered by this license would not lead to penalties on the main laboratory.

We initiated a strategy to develop a second license and director under which all the laboratories in the second category and some of those in the first would be covered.

Affiliated Laboratories

University Health Service.— The laboratory serving the student body of the University of Wisconsin was not associated with the laboratory at the university hospital. University Health Services was about 1 mile from UWHC. University Health Services began to restructure, and its new director, Richard Keeling, MD, asked if we would be interested in some arrangement concerning the laboratory. After only a few meetings, it was clear that University Health Services had two objectives—get out of the laboratory business and save money. After reviewing the budget, personnel, workload, etc, from the facility, we recognized that we could not only perform their procedures more economically but also provide a higher quality of service in turnaround-time, menu, consultations, and computer reports. The plan was presented to UWHC hospital administration, which supported the concept and the specifics. Hospital administration asked only that the laboratory effort not be a financial drain on the hospital. After several more months of contract building and reviews within each organization and the state bureaucracy, an agreement was signed and the University Health Services Laboratory became a UWHC Clinical Laboratory. We offered positions to the personnel at University Health Services and eventually rotated most of the employees through the University of Wisconsin laboratories in the specimen control section. Through cross-training and increased efficiencies at University Health Services, we were able to maintain the same number of total employees in the laboratory. Thus, we added a new service without adding new position lines and integrated the three employees from University Health Services into our structure.

We added a new service without adding new position lines.

Hospital-Initiated Laboratories.—Beginning in 1988, UWHC underwent a series of expansionist moves to increase its flow of patients. Because space at the main building was not available, the first move was to open a set of specialty clinics about a block from the hospital. The facility housing the clinics is called University Station. Ophthalmology, Mohs' chemosurgery, and many of the subspecialties of internal medicine moved to this facility in 1989. Support diagnostic facilities, ie, radiology and clinical laboratory, are available within University Station and under the control of the hospital. The University Station Laboratory was an extension of UWHC with full integration of its policies, procedures, and personnel. Nevertheless, by law, the laboratory required a separate license.

As the population level of the east side of Madison increased, the leadership of UWHC perceived and their practice plans reflected the need to develop an "east side" presence. After some discussion and analysis of need and costs, the clinicians at the newly conceived "University East Clinic" agreed to perform only phlebotomy and wavered testing onsite. Other testing was forwarded to the main laboratory. Computers were installed at the east side clinic to allow the rapid tracking and reporting of laboratory data. While at first only a pilot study, the east side clinic staff agreed that the level of laboratory service met its needs. This clinic is also part of UWHC and its laboratory activities were also integrated into the main laboratory.

Nonhospital Initiated Laboratories.—Two other offsite laboratories were also supported by the central laboratory, but with somewhat different arrangements. The sports medicine program had been offsite for several years but had been growing and needed larger quarters. In the fall of 1995, a new building was opened that housed an expanded sports medicine program. Within this facility, a three-person family practice was also housed. This group felt it needed a laboratory and because it rented the space from UWHC, it was considered a family practice laboratory. We were asked to consult about the menu, personnel, space, and design of this laboratory. After a review of needs and costs, the clinicians agreed to perform only phlebotomy and wavered tests onsite. All other testing was sent to UWHC at discounted testing rates.

The last clinic was one opened on the west side of Madison by the department of medicine and clinical practice groups of the University of Wisconsin. We were asked to comment on the planned laboratory operations. Unfortunately, menus had been set, equipment purchased, and budgeted lines finalized. There was also no provision for computer support. From the data shared with us, it became apparent that many cost items had been ignored, including inspection, accreditation, licensure, preventive maintenance, etc. The net revenues were also greatly overestimated. UWHC acted only as an informal consultant to this effort. The clinic opened and was not profitable and in fact, could not pay its laboratory fees. UWHC eventually became more involved with the management of the facility to help maintain its financial integrity.

UWHC as a Reference Laboratory

Many of the patients receiving treatment at UWHC require "tertiary care," ie, treatment programs not generally available in community hospitals. These programs include the transplantation programs, the trauma and burn units, and the cancer center with its multiple treatment protocols. Such "cutting-edge" programs require a state-of-the-art support structure, including clinical laboratory facilities. The laboratory is expected to provide a large menu of determinations available in a timely fashion, often at any time of the day or week. The clinical services require rapid turnaround-times that preclude "outsourcing" most assays that otherwise would not be available in this community. Because we were required to have a higher expertise than the other laboratories in the area, we aimed to use this to our advantage, to attract testing from other local and regional sources. We initiated this strategy in several ways.

Between a Rock and a Hard Place; Preparing Proposals.—By 1988, the UWHC Clinical Laboratory culture had turned inward, ie, taking care of in-patients well but paying little heed to the samples it received from external sources. Thus, because of its lack of interest and neglect, UWHC received relatively few test requests from other community providers. Reference samples that might have been done at UWHC were sent to out-of-state facilities, and there was little interest within the laboratory in attracting these samples. Further, we were aware that several hospital services were either substandard or nonexistent and would need to be addressed for us to be competitive. Specifically, this included courier and billing services. In fact, we lost our first external account

From the data shared with us, it became apparent that many cost items had been ignored, including inspection, accreditation, licensure, preventive maintenance, etc. The net revenues were also greatly overestimated.

We were aware that several hospital services were either substandard or nonexistent and would need to be addressed for us to be competitive.

because of inaccurate, incomplete billing. These issues were discussed with hospital administration many times but were never completely resolved. The billing services remained unsatisfactory, and the laboratory was not given the responsibility of managing these areas directly.

It seemed clear, however, that the laboratory had the talent and capacity to serve as a reference laboratory for and in collaboration with community facilities. It was in UWHC's long-term interests to maintain our specialty testing but to reduce the cost per assay by increasing samples. It was in the interest of the other laboratories to have a local site with specialty capability with the caveat that the service provided had to be excellent and the charges competitive. We established project teams with different hospital administrative elements to address the major concerns. An improvement in courier services resulted from these efforts.

The laboratory had never prepared a formal proposal for reference testing. Each year, several groups sent UWHC requests for proposals. It was not until we were well into our total quality management (TQM) and outreach educational efforts and had the availability of an outreach supervisor that we could put together a competitive proposal. This was done for the Wisconsin Department of Family Medicine's laboratories that were located throughout the state of Wisconsin. Although the Department of Family Medicine evaluation committee rated our proposal number one, the members of the department felt uncomfortable moving from its existing laboratory, which was in its primary hospital, not UWHC. Because members of the Department of Family Medicine had only recently been able to admit and care for patients at UWHC, their loyalty remained with the community hospital. We were advised to try again when the contracts would be renewed, perhaps 3 to 5 years in the future.

While we were not successful, several positives arose from this effort. First, we learned how to put together a proposal, including the operations and financial sections; we sent a message to the laboratory that we were serious about becoming a reference site; we learned much more about the laboratory community beyond UWHC; and we learned that being the best did not guarantee success in this highly competitive, political arena.

We learned how to put together a proposal, including the operations and financial sections; we sent a message to the laboratory that we were serious about becoming a reference site.

Discussions With Other City Laboratories

The State Laboratory of Hygiene.—The Wisconsin State Laboratory of Hygiene (SLH) and the UWHC Clinical Laboratory have had an ambivalent relationship. SLH was organizationally part of the University of Wisconsin and physically on the campus, across a parking lot from the medical school and 1.5 miles from the hospital. Its director, medical director, and associate medical director held academic positions in the department of pathology and laboratory medicine, the academic home of all the professional staff in the UWHC Clinical Laboratory. We shared several teaching and research activities. However, SLH performed many "routine" laboratory assays for physicians in the state. In addition, it performed many more specialized tests. While these were fee-for-service, they were subsidized and often priced below the laboratory market and even laboratory costs. Thus, while we were able to use the locally available specialized testing, we were discouraged from establishing our own specialized testings.

However, SLH was under pressure to reduce costs and to redefine its mission. More specifically, it was not to duplicate services available in the private sector. SLH was to focus on public health needs. The SLH director and the UWHC Clinical Laboratory director both believed that cooperation between their units would be mutually beneficial. Thus, a series of meetings were held among the directors and their senior administrators. These focused on the overlapping menus, volumes, and courier and computer services. A plan was developed to consolidate some areas of services in one or the other laboratories, consider developing a third entity for external reference work, and enhance courier services. Some of these efforts were carried out. Unfortunately for both units, most of the plans were not completed. The reasons for this incomplete success are complex; however, the prime reason, at least to the UWHC team, seemed to be the inability of SLH administrators to implement the plans. For example, it was agreed that immunology testing, especially anti-nuclear antibody, would be moved eventually to UWHC. This was to occur after other plans had been implemented. However, shortly after this agreement, SLH announced that it was closing its immunology testing. The UWHC Clinical Laboratory was among the last to know of this development!

General Medical Laboratory.—General Medical Laboratory (GML) was a semi-independent laboratory of a community not-for-profit hospital, Meriter-Madison. UWHC performed some reference testing for GML but there had been little communication or cooperation between the laboratories. We were concerned about maintaining and even increasing reference testing from GML. We also wondered if there might be other mutually beneficial opportunities. Thus, the UWHC Clinical Laboratory director and a senior hospital administrator met with senior laboratory and hospital administrators at GML. We explored possible areas of cooperation and started a series of meetings that led to reduced reference rates for GML and increased reference test volume for UWHC. We had agreed to investigate menus and volumes to determine if tests might be done at either site rather than an external reference laboratory and if the combined volumes of send-outs might be sufficient to either establish the assay in town or reduce the external reference charges though an improved negotiating position. Finally, we raised the issue of further consolidation.

Specialty Testing at UWHC.—The UWHC Clinical Laboratory once had been a leader in development of laboratory technology. While it remained competent, it was no longer exceptional. The laboratory, however, performed some determinations that still attracted local or regional attention and requests for testing. Specialized testing in the immunology laboratory, directed by Richard Hong, MD, was the most requested. These came from other pediatric immunologists to help diagnose and manage immunodeficiency disorders and to support experimental therapies such as bone marrow and thymus transplantation. Some requests for analysis of trace elements were directed toward a unit developed by Merle Evenson, PhD. The special coagulation laboratory, directed by Dean Moser, MD, and Elliot Williams, MD received local requests for sophisticated testing. At times, the toxicology unit received special requests for analysis of unknown or atypical analytes.

One of the efforts at bringing the clinical laboratory back to the "cutting edge" of analysis was the establishment of a molecular diagnostic section. The first research physician hired by the laboratory director was charged with development of this important area. Administratively, this section was placed in a larger area, called special chemistry, so that its costs could be absorbed by a "profit center." In time, a second technologist and a second professional, a PhD with a background in molecular biology, were added. Molecular diagnosis training is critical for house staff, medical technologists, and support of the tertiary care programs in the medical center as well as the pride of the members of the laboratory and department. The positions other than that of the physician were not "new" but transferred and upgraded slots from other units.

To complement this effort, we were able to name a new director of tissue typing (histocompatibility). The opportunity developed as the university's primate center sought a researcher with an excellent molecular biology approach to nonhuman primate histocompatibility. With the cooperation of the department of pathology and laboratory medicine, hospital administration, and the political support of the section of transplantation surgery, we were able to develop a tenured home position in the department of pathology and laboratory medicine with research space and support in the primate center. This person rapidly brought molecular diagnostics to histocompatibility.

When the time came to hire a new director of hematopathology, we sought someone who would bring "added value" to our missions. The person who was hired brought with him expertise in flow cytometry and immunohistochemistry, thus strengthening two important areas of specialized testing.

It was apparent that the laboratory needed additional direction on development of new assays. Each section had somewhat different priorities and each had variable resources. Finances dictated that a more studied approach would be required. As a beginning, the laboratory director encouraged the formation of a development group that would meet to discuss goals, priorities, and resources in each of their sections. Thus, the developmental group began meeting monthly. It had immediate positive effects as technologies and skills were shared to induce the more rapid development of several assays. The technologists were far less controlling of their turf than the section directors or supervisors. Thus, empowering the "research and development" technologists led to a more cooperative, productive effort. Further, from this group came the development of a less expensive, more accurate assay for cyclosporine, one of our biggest supply budget items. In a similar manner, an assay for gabapentin was also developed.

While hospital administration voiced support for research and development, it did not readily provide the necessary resources. Only after 4 years of promises and negotiation was the laboratory given $100,000/year to spend on research and development. We soon discovered, however, that this money could not be readily used for personnel or capital equipment but only for supplies, which had to be requested through the usual hospital reviews and bidding processes. Attempts to free the funds from these constraints failed. Nevertheless, with perseverance, the funds were eventually used to establish an assay for plasma HIV-1 RNA. Personnel was made available through the developmental group, and a reagent rental agreement provided the necessary equipment.

Each of the sections was thus encouraged to consider reference testing, by reviewing send-outs to determine if it would improve service and/or economics to bring testing in-house.

The Marketing Group.—The technologists who developed cyclosporine and gabapentin assays pointed out that these and perhaps other tests might be marketed by our laboratory to external sources. We requested help from hospital administration and a team was put together to develop a process for marketing our products (see appendix). With the help of Bill Nitzke from hospital administration, we began to put together a strategy and a brochure to let others know of our capabilities.

Medical Advisory Group

The lines of communication between the medical staff and the clinical laboratory were, for the most part, informal and uneven. There existed no recurring procedure for the laboratory to obtain clinical input or for the medical staff to voice its concerns, complaints, or compliments about the laboratory. The laboratory director began to address these needs by attempting to form a medical advisory group that was to meet monthly to discuss issues of mutual interest to the laboratory and the

While hospital administration voiced support for research and development, it did not readily provide the necessary resources.

medical staff. The laboratory director asked the chairs of the departments who used the laboratory the most, ie, surgery, medicine, pediatrics, etc, to name a representative to the medical advisory committee. This committee had no official recognition by the medical board and was only advisory to the laboratory director. The members appointed by the chairs did not have sufficient interest to regularly attend the monthly meetings and the effort soon died. The group was reformulated in late 1991 at which time the laboratory director openly approached a group of physicians who he knew had some special interest in the laboratory—either by acting as a laboratory consultant or requiring some unusual services. Dr Richard Hong (pediatrics) was the first chair of the committee, followed by John Pirsch, MD (medicine and transplantation surgery), and William Perloff, MD (pediatrics and intensive care).

The laboratory director openly approached a group of physicians who he knew had some special interest in the laboratory.

The committee's mission is to provide guidance to the clinical laboratory on the quality of patient care issues. This includes choices among services to provide, methods of data reporting, incorporation of consultative roles, quality requirement definitions for laboratory services, and methods of continuing education for hospital personnel.

During the first sessions, a laundry list of outstanding items was developed through brainstorming by the committee membership. Most of the items involved communication problems. The supervisor of data processing was asked to attend the committee meetings regularly and begin to address these issues. These problems existed primarily because the laboratory was not aware that they were problems; however, once they were brought into the open, most were easily resolved. Encouraged by its success, the committee continued its efforts and began moving into more complex areas.

Most of the items involved communication problems.

These problems existed primarily because the laboratory was not aware that they were problems.

Some of the agenda items during the next 4 years included the direction and support of molecular diagnostics, the development of a liver panel, review and rewriting of critical values for each laboratory section, review and standardization of prewritten orders for the medical center, discussions about laboratory utilization and education of medical staff, and changes in some reporting procedures. In each item, at least one positive step was implemented to create an improvement in the previous practice.

Eventually, all the laboratory section directors and some of the supervisors attended the Medical Advisory Committee meetings. This provided a time and place for dialogue between the laboratory and the clinical staff. Attempts by the laboratory director to have this group recognized formally by the hospital were unsuccessful.

Union Cooperation

The Wisconsin Science Professionals (WSP), an arm of the Wisconsin Teachers Union, represented most of the technologists in the UWHC

Clinical Laboratory. Clerical workers, dishwashers, and medical laboratory technicians (MLT) were represented by another union, the Wisconsin State Employees Union (WSEU). Supervisory staff were considered "nonrepresented professionals." Although "academic staff" and faculty each had professional organizations, these units did no contractual bargaining. Thus, contracts, work rules, policies, and procedures for 85% of the laboratory employees were negotiated between the WSP and the State of Wisconsin Department of Employee Relations (DER). While the hospital and thus the laboratory had input into the biennial bargaining process, it did not deal directly with the union. On its part, the WSP representatives did not necessarily include anyone from the UWHC Clinical Laboratory.

Soon after the UWHC Clinical Laboratory director was appointed, he began to encourage a beneficial relationship with the union by maintaining communication between union representatives and the laboratory administration. Further, he requested union advice before proceeding with programs that might alter the expectations of union members. Overall, the relationship with the union was open and cooperative.

Union cooperation was imperative if reengineering were to be successful. Over the years, job descriptions had become very specific. In fact, the rules were written so specifically that job titles could be changed only by agreement of all involved employees or by firing everyone and rehiring them into new classifications with new job descriptions! This was actually done at another university clinical laboratory in the Midwest. We viewed such a course of action as a catastrophic failure of management. We needed to change and increase flexibility by cross-training and cross-coverage. We aimed to accomplish any required downsizing through attrition. In addition, we wanted to maintain the option of hiring those with special training and skills to enhance our development of "cutting edge" assays.

In the winter and spring of 1994, the laboratory director and the senior laboratory manager first met with the laboratory's past and present union representatives to hear their concerns and eventually to enlist their support. After these informal contacts, the director and senior laboratory manager drafted a proposal for consideration by the union. We asked the laboratory union representatives and then other employees to review this document. At the same time, we requested hospital administration, ie, human resources and the senior administrator with responsibility for the laboratory, to review the proposal. After a series of redrafts, all parties agreed to the document's language and intent.

The group then came together comprising of representatives of the WSP, the Wisconsin State Teachers Union, the UWHC Clinical Laboratory, and UWHC human resources. The draft was presented and

Union cooperation was imperative if reengineering were to be successful.

discussed. After the concerns and acceptable solutions were aired, each representative was asked to comment formally on the draft, which was then rewritten and accepted by all parties in the winter of 1995. This was to be considered a draft of understanding until it was formally incorporated into the new union-DER contract to be finalized in 1996.

The completion of this agreement removed what could have been a major hurdle.

The completion of this agreement removed what could have been a major hurdle in reengineering in that it provided a process for cross-training and moving employees into other areas such as a core laboratory.

External Consultation

Dr Larry Maguire had been a participant in our Automations Workshop Program held in Madison in 1993. Although an internist/hematologist, Dr Maguire became interested in laboratory automation, specifically sample processing. He formed a company, Medical Robotics, and began to market his innovations. During his interactions with laboratorians and administrators, he recognized the need to analyze systems and their processes, rather than just a single element within the system. Thus, he joined forces with an industrial consulting firm, Belcan Engineering Group, to offer consultative services to clinical laboratories.

Belcan Engineering Group was spun off from an internal consultative group within the Procter & Gamble Company. Its processes incorporated both TQM and Hammer and Champy's reengineering. Belcan Engineering Group was aligned with a manufacturing firm, Process Equipment of Dayton, which could "make" laboratory instruments, as needed.

At the conclusion of the Automations Workshop, Dr Maguire proposed a brief, 3-day Belcan review of the reengineering program at the UWHC Clinical Laboratory. The cost of this would be minimal. We would then have the option of going on with a more detailed program, hiring Belcan Engineering as an external consultant and facilitating agent for reengineering. An implementation phase would then follow the planning period.

Dr Maguire formally made his proposal in June 1993. We believed that an external review would help the laboratory by critiquing our plans and progress and add insights from an organization experienced in consultation and automation manufacturing. We also believed that our discussions with hospital administration would be strengthened by an outside reviewer. We needed to obtain funds from the hospital to proceed. The meeting with Belcan Engineering finally took place in April 1994.

Before arriving in Madison, Belcan Engineering asked for some input and specifically what we expected from the consultants. Belcan Engineering asked for this in the form of a mission statement. Such a statement was drafted by the laboratory director after discussions with hospital administration and senior laboratory members. We listed the following four "jobs" for an external consultant:

1. Review and assess our existing documentation of systems in the clinical laboratories as a baseline for planning activities.

2. Recommend a plan to optimize high quality, efficient laboratory services.

3. Provide a cost-benefit analysis of this plan.

4. Propose a process for the plan's implementation.

About 2 weeks before its visit, Belcan Engineering sent a proposed schedule, prework materials, a proposed structure for the team to meet with Belcan, and described the role of the Belcan consultants.

Four members of the Belcan Engineering team arrived Wednesday evening, April 6, 1994, with sessions to start the next day. After a laboratory tour, presentations were made by each of the laboratory sections that we believed would be involved in the initial phases of reengineering. Most of Friday was spent in a workshop conducted by Belcan Engineering with selected laboratory personnel. Belcan Engineering representatives then spent the weekend reviewing the information and formulating their findings, which were presented Monday morning to the clinical laboratory's reengineering team. After clarifications, a discussion of the findings ensued before the Belcan team left Madison.

The consultative report consisted of four parts:

1. Review of the Belcan Total Quality Reengineering methodology

2. The learnings gathered from the data generated by the laboratory and the visit

3. Recommendations for next steps

4. An assessment of the clinical laboratory's recommendations

Belcan Engineering's recommendations were organized into the five segments it uses to help define total quality reengineering—qualities, processes, organization, systems, and operations. Overall, these focused on the continuance of TQM in the laboratory, development and implementation of strategic planning, expansion of influence within the hospital and medical center, and expansion of outreach efforts. The following is an abridged version of 24 discrete recommendations.

Belcan Engineering reviewed the 21 recommendations made by the clinical laboratory team (see Table 3-1). It sorted these into five components, quality, process, organization, systems, and operations, before noting its opinion of a specific recommendation. Belcan

Engineering agreed with only 10 of the 21 recommendations made by the clinical laboratory team. There was general agreement on what needed to be done but not on the specific methods, particularly changes in organization structure, suggested by the internal group. For example, Belcan Engineering agreed with the recommendations to reevaluate quality requirements for patient care including POC testing but not with the specifics of organizing the laboratory into four managerial segments. The consulting group believed that organizational changes should follow process rather than be imposed at the outset.

The clinical laboratory director had come to the same conclusions and had obtained similar views from colleagues in industrial management; however, those who had worked so hard on the internal report were concerned that Belcan Engineering had not spent sufficient time to justify its recommendations. Because it would have been difficult, if not impossible, to obtain funding for further consultation, the decision was made to proceed internally without external support. However, the lessons learned from Belcan Engineering were incorporated into the formation of a Reengineering Implementation Steering Committee (RISC), which was to supervise the implementation of laboratory restructuring.

The Reengineering Implementation Steering Committee (RISC)

ESTABLISHING GROUND RULES

The laboratory was now prepared to engage on its adventure of reengineering. Faculty and staff were at worst neutral and at best enthusiastic; hospital administration was cautiously supportive; the department of pathology and laboratory medicine was silent; the medical school was disinterested. We needed an administrative team to oversee the implementation of reengineering, particularly to have the power to deal with problems and potential obstacles as they arose. This team was called the Reengineering Implementation Steering Committee (RISC).

We had learned that the two critical features required to enhance the chances for a successful project team were a well-defined mission and the team's composition.

The mission was not difficult. The laboratory director, with review by some senior laboratory staff, suggested the following:

The two critical features required to enhance the chances for a successful project team were a well-defined mission and the team's composition.

- Decide what needs to be done.

- Develop a timetable for reengineering.

- Assign tasks.

- Monitor and facilitate the reengineering process.

The Belcan Engineering consultants had suggested that we include all the interested parties in our planning teams. We set out to accomplish this goal in selecting the membership of the RISC. We named four laboratory members of the faculty—the laboratory director, associate director, director of data processing, and director of quality assurance. These individuals had been most involved with the earlier planning. We added a fifth faculty member, the director of clinical chemistry, because this section would be most affected by the development of a core laboratory. The senior laboratory manager represented the technical staff and also had been involved in the earlier planning. Two senior hospital administrators were recruited and accepted membership. One was the administrator most involved in the daily laboratory operations; the other was responsible for human resources, an area we perceived as potentially the most contentious in implementing reengineering. We asked for representatives from the dean's office and the office of the chair of pathology and laboratory medicine. We received no reply to our inquiries.

The first meeting was held on December 19, 1994, at which time we reviewed and accepted the mission and established RISC ground rules. These rules were (1) the 100-mile rule: there would be no interruptions and we would behave as if we were 100 miles from our place of work; (2) we defined a quorum as five for a meeting to be held but that no decision would be made on a key issue in the absence of a key person (as defined by the Chair); (3) we would meet weekly for 1-1/2 hours at first; (4) we might require a retreat to consolidate findings; (5) all members would be expected to participate; (6) meetings would start and end on time.

The committee was presented a summary of past activities and provided an opportunity to ask questions about the previous work.

The most critical item for reengineering was the formation of a core laboratory.

RISC fully agreed that the most critical item for reengineering was the formation of a core laboratory and that we should focus on that project.

The team proposed that a facilitator be named and one of the hospital administrators suggested an experienced person in the hospital quality assurance program. This suggestion was accepted.

We determined that at the next meeting we would begin to define what needed to be done to form a core laboratory.

WHAT DO WE NEED TO DO FOR THE CORE LABORATORY TO OCCUR?
Brainstorming and Affinity Diagram

The laboratory director met with the newly named team facilitator before the team meeting. This pattern continued throughout the process and was critical to advancing the project.

The objective of our first facilitated session was to identify those factors necessary to implement a core laboratory. We followed the now familiar process of brainstorming, asking each person in turn for his or her suggestions on this topic until there were no further ideas. The facilitator wrote these on Post-it® Notes (3M, St Paul, Minn) and placed them randomly on flip charts. We then asked for clarification of the terms to be sure that there was a common understanding of the suggestions. Finally, each team member was asked to come to the flip charts and independently group the Post-it Notes by their affinity to one another. This continued until the team came to a consensus about the arrangement. The facilitator recorded the final grouping and sent copies to the team members asking for changes in arrangement or wordings or additions to the items to be discussed at the next meeting.

Interrelationship Diagraph

The brainstorming and affinity diagram included 10 broad categories with several items under each category (Figure 5-1). The team discussed and agreed on a final version of the affinity diagram and next embarked on prioritizing the items. We used an interrelationship diagraph for this purpose. On a 10 × 10 grid, each item was listed along the top as well as on the left-hand side. Team members were asked to consider if an item was the cause or the effect of each of the other items on the chart. We discussed each of the 10 items and decided to remove 2 of them—1 dealt with finances and politics because it was beyond the responsibility of our team and because we already had reassurances of support, and the other dealt with issues to consider after a core laboratory was formed. The team quickly came to a consensus in assigning cause ("out") or effect ("in") or both ("out" and "in") for each of the remaining items (Figure 5-2). Defining the boundaries of the core laboratory was the overwhelming "winner," ie, having an effect on all other items. Our next sessions focused on what tests were to be included in the core laboratory.

COMMUNICATIONS

As RISC was beginning its work, the laboratory director met with all members of the laboratory staff to discuss the prospective changes, process, and progress of the reengineering project. Thus, twelve 30- to 60-minute meetings were held during a 3-week period to allow for presentations and open discussions of the laboratory's future. Supervisors had been asked to schedule their staff to ensure opportunity for all members to attend one of the sessions. In addition, RISC had begun to post its meeting minutes so that all staff would have access. Laboratory staff were encouraged to speak with one or more of the RISC members if they had specific questions or concerns. Much of this was done using the laboratory's e-mail system or informally throughout the unit.

DEFINING THE CORE LABORATORY

A previous team had suggested criteria for inclusion in the core laboratory and suggested a first approximation of which tests should be included, which should be excluded, and which were on-the-bubble.

The information was provided to RISC and discussed in some detail. Each member then reviewed both the core laboratory inclusion criteria and the test lists with other laboratory staff before the next meeting. We were particularly interested in comments on the assays that were not so obviously included or excluded from the core laboratory.

At the next two meetings, the criteria for inclusion and the specific measurements to be included were reviewed until all members of RISC were satisfied with the result. The criteria for inclusion were a 24-

Figure 5-1.
This diagram was developed by brainstorming and then gathering similar functions together in an affinity diagram.

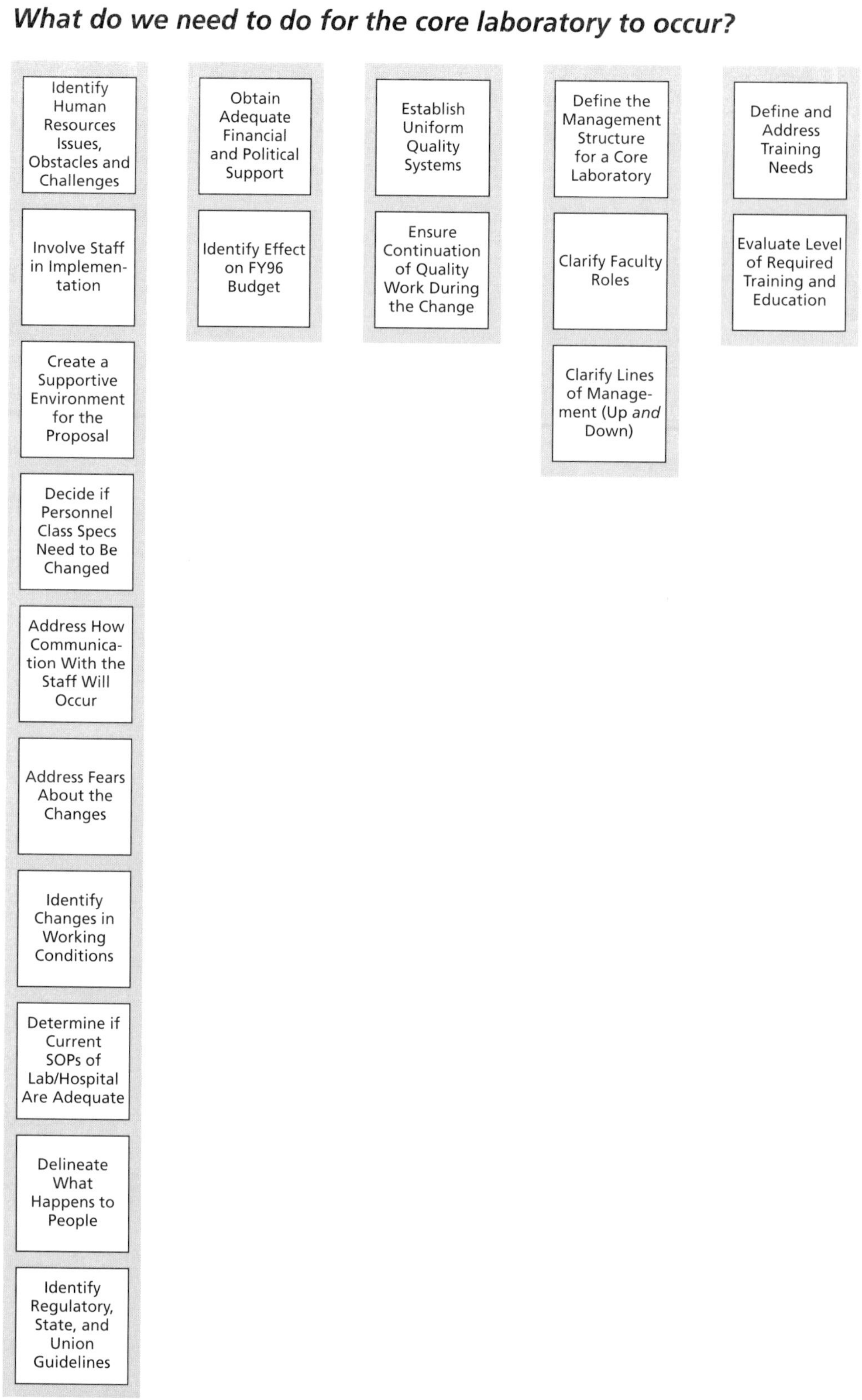

What do we need to do for the core laboratory to occur?

Identify Human Resources Issues, Obstacles and Challenges	Obtain Adequate Financial and Political Support	Establish Uniform Quality Systems	Define the Management Structure for a Core Laboratory	Define and Address Training Needs
Involve Staff in Implementation	Identify Effect on FY96 Budget	Ensure Continuation of Quality Work During the Change	Clarify Faculty Roles	Evaluate Level of Required Training and Education
Create a Supportive Environment for the Proposal			Clarify Lines of Management (Up *and* Down)	
Decide if Personnel Class Specs Need to Be Changed				
Address How Communication With the Staff Will Occur				
Address Fears About the Changes				
Identify Changes in Working Conditions				
Determine if Current SOPs of Lab/Hospital Are Adequate				
Delineate What Happens to People				
Identify Regulatory, State, and Union Guidelines				

Develop a Remodeling Plan	Instrument Resources	Empower, Facilitate, and Monitor Project Teams	Define the Boundaries of the Core Laboratory	Determine Relationship of Other Parts of Lab to Core Laboratory
Address Noise Level as Remodeling Is Done	Insure Current Bids Select the *Right* Instruments	Monitor, Co-ordinate On-going Changes to Ensure Consistency With Core Lab	Define Criteria for Evaluating Success of Core Laboratory	Look at Specimen Transporta-tion Issue
Identify Facility Modifications	Acquire New Equipment Not Present, but Needed	Establish a Do-it Team	Identify Anticipated Service Improvements	Decide What Nursing Unit Bar Coding Is Needed
	Move Equipment		Define Role of Heme Lab	Determine if There Will be Additional Needs for Computer Support
	Evaluation of Present Instrument and Work Stations		Identify all Initial Components of Core Laboratory	Decide How Outreach and Reference Work Fits Into Core Laboratory
			Establish a Time Line	
			Review Current Plans for Core Laboratory	

Figure 5-2.
An interrelationship diagraph was developed using the eight processes required to develop a core laboratory. Each item was reviewed individually to determine if it had a cause-or-effect relationship with each of the other items. For example, column 4 (instrument resources) had an effect on row 1 (human resource issues) but was itself affected by row 2 (establish uniform quality system). Arrows were summarized and are designated as "IN" or "OUT" on the right side of the graph.

	1	2	3	4	5	6	7	8	In	Out	Total
1. ID Human Resource Issues									6	4	**10**
2. Establish Uniform Quality System									2	5	7
3. Define and Address Training Needs									5	2	7
4. Instrument Resources									2	4	6
5. Define Boundaries of Core Lab									1	7	8
6. Define Management Structure for a Core Lab									2	3	5
7. Develop a Remodeling Plan									2	2	4
8. Finalize Plans; Establish Time Lines; Empower, Facilitate, and Monitor Project Teams									7	0	7

hour/day service; automated processes available; cross-training feasible; rapid turnaround-time/stat needed; high volume; continuous monitoring required; moderate complexity or less as defined by CLIA; physical safety facilities adequate. We realized that not all tests needed to meet all these criteria. The final test lists are given in Table 4-1.

HUMAN RESOURCES, INSTRUMENTATION, UNIFORM QUALITY SYSTEMS

As we discussed the components of the core laboratory, we began to prepare to make decisions about the next three items from our original list of tasks required to implement a core laboratory. We assigned three subgroups to review the current status, potential opportunities and obstacles in human resources, instrumentation, and uniform quality systems. These items had received the most "cause" votes after defining the core laboratory in our interrelationship diagraph (Figure 5-2). Considerable effort already had been made in each of these areas, and those individuals most involved in the process were asked to update the other RISC members.

At RISC's next meeting, we heard the director of quality assurance report on his group's efforts in ensuring uniform quality systems in the core laboratory, ie, that specific policies and procedures could now be written because the core laboratory menu was nearly finalized. In subsequent sessions, the directors of clinical chemistry and data processing shared their lists of instruments to be included in the core laboratory. They also included the lease or ownership and age status of each instrument as well as its test menu, throughput, and automation capacities (bar coding characteristics, random access capabilities, etc). Finally, the laboratory director, senior laboratory manager, and hospital associate superintendent responsible for human resources reviewed the status of contractual union agreements, memoranda of understanding, and State of Wisconsin administrative codes. From these reports, the members of RISC agreed that we were prepared to begin the next phases of reengineering.

We recognized that physical remodeling of our current space would almost surely be required and that planning, financing, and implementing such a program would be critical if the core laboratory were to become functional in the near future. Thus, the laboratory director named a remodeling team or space team that included members from the hospital planning sections along with RISC and laboratory staff members and the microbiology supervisor, who was also chair. The space team frequently consulted with the hospital's physical plant section. The remodeling team was to develop a plan based on the core laboratory assays plus our previous work on space use. It was to develop a

We recognized that physical remodeling of our current space would almost surely be required and that planning, financing, and implementing such a program would be critical.

time frame for the completion of remodeling as well as provide a more exact cost estimate. The core laboratory assays were classified by work station to help guide the remodeling plans.

At this point, we knew the tests, instruments, and work stations to be included in the core laboratory. We had cross-training teams working for more than 2 years, initially to help staff the third shift more completely, but later to learn how best to go about the business of increasing the scope of our technologists' activities while maintaining quality. We asked the team leader, a supervisor in clinical chemistry, to lead a group to look into core laboratory staffing issues.

The laboratory director met with both the space and staffing teams to deliver their charges and respond to questions. The teams were directed to communicate openly with each other, RISC, and the rest of the laboratory orally and through e-mail. Minutes were to be posted for all to read. We asked the space team to draft a plan for the core laboratory based on the existing plan, gather data as needed, provide some time lines and cost estimates, and report to RISC in 4 weeks.

The staffing team was directed to determine the number and type of bench level staffing required for each shift in the core laboratory; determine training requirements; and comment on back-up, scheduling, and if time permitted, supervision. We asked that it report to RISC in 6 weeks. A series of specific questions to be answered, developed by the laboratory director and reviewed by several senior laboratory administrators, was given to each team.

THE REPORT FROM THE SPACE TEAM

The principles for redesigning space were (1) installation of a transport system that would record specimens (through bar coding) and move samples to work stations; (2) consolidation of workstations; (3) stratification of chemistry analyzers by stat, profiling, and "unusual testing"; (4) reduction and apposition of workstations to facilitate cross-coverage; and (5) reduction of redundant methods and instruments. A drawing of the space team's recommended layout is given in Figure 5-3F. For comparison, earlier stages of planning are represented in Figures 5-3A–E.

During its deliberations, the team recognized three areas that required more study and suggested that subgroups be appointed to gather data and make recommendations on (1) record storage and retrieval, (2) refrigerator and freezer storage, and (3) the effect on the laboratory's educational programs.

THE REPORT FROM THE STAFFING TEAM

The staffing team used the workstation configuration developed by the space team (infra vide) plus the experience gained in cross-training and

Figure 5-3A.
A. The layout of the laboratory prior to any changes. **B.** A conceptual proposal from the first reengineering team, September 1993. **C.** An approach proposed by the instrumentation team, January 1994. **D.** The first attempt to adopt concepts to the physical space provided by the transport and storage team, February 1994. **E.** More details added by the cost/benefit team, September 1994. **F.** The final version drafted by the space team of the reengineering implementation steering team, May 1995. Chem Anal = chemical analyzer; Endo Drug = endocrinology and drug testing; SSI = setup, storage, and information; DIFF Station = differential station.

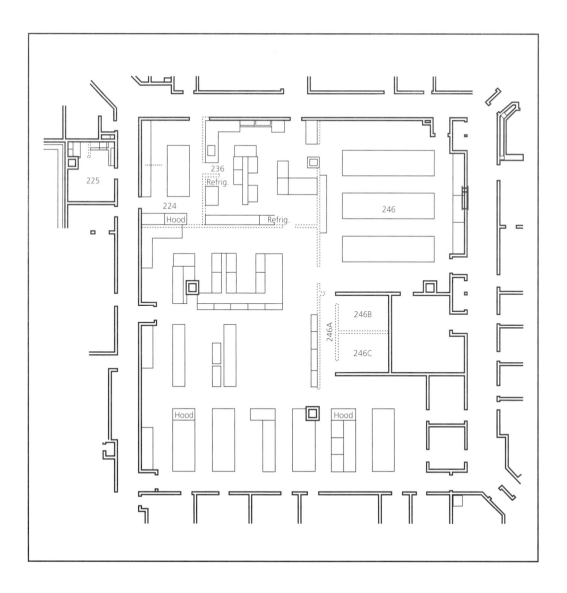

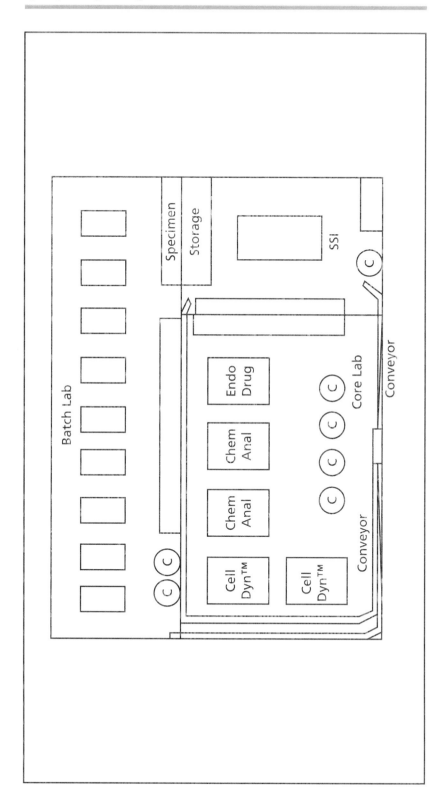

Figure 5-3B.

Figure 5-3C.

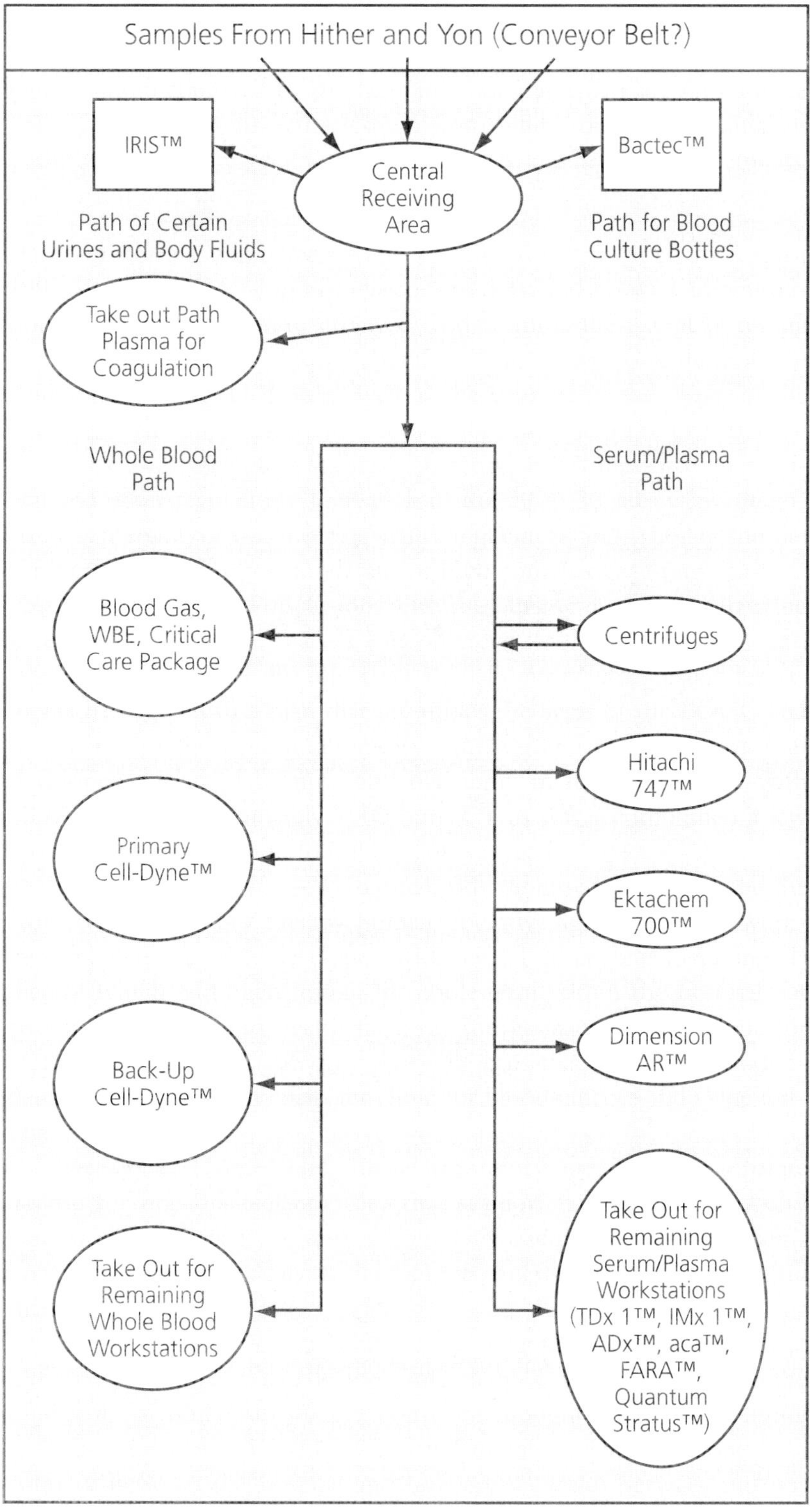
Samples From Hither and Yon (Conveyor Belt?)
IRIS™
Central Receiving Area
Bactec™
Path of Certain Urines and Body Fluids
Path for Blood Culture Bottles
Take out Path Plasma for Coagulation
Whole Blood Path
Serum/Plasma Path
Blood Gas, WBE, Critical Care Package
Centrifuges
Hitachi 747™
Primary Cell-Dyne™
Ektachem 700™
Dimension AR™
Back-Up Cell-Dyne™
Take Out for Remaining Whole Blood Workstations
Take Out for Remaining Serum/Plasma Workstations (TDx 1™, IMx 1™, ADx™, aca™, FARA™, Quantum Stratus™)

Figure 5-3D.

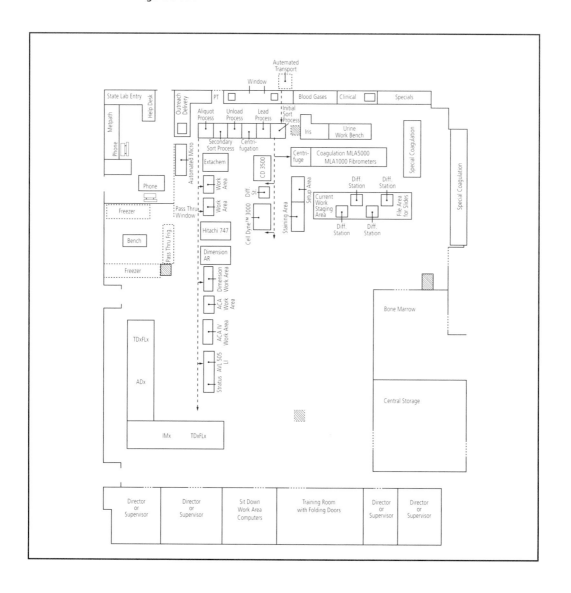

Figure 5-3E.

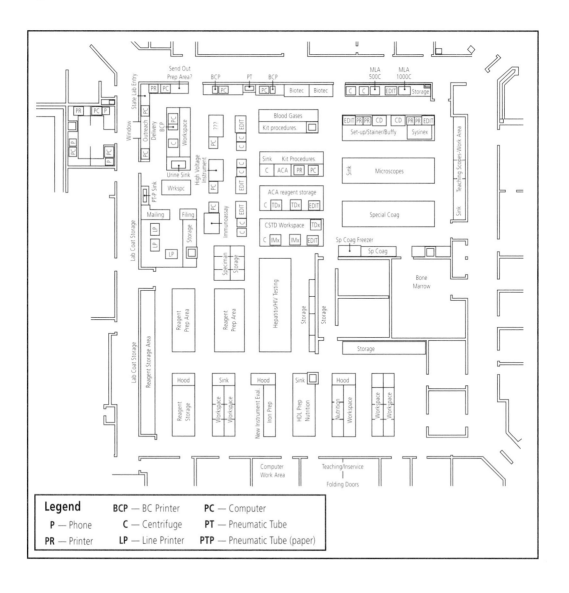

Figure 5-3F.

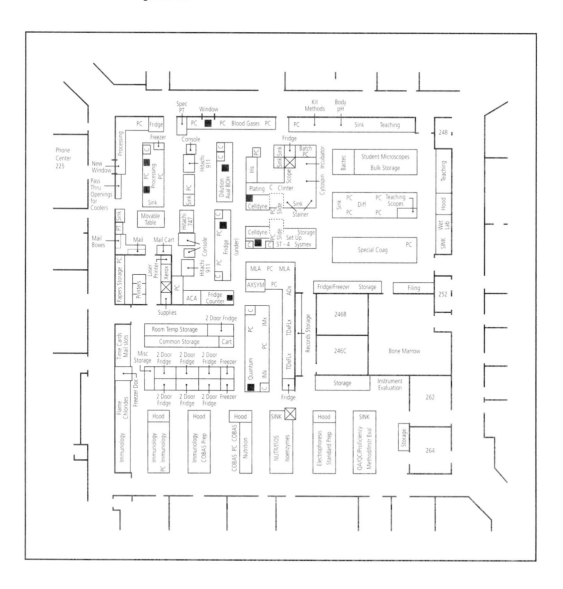

cross-coverage for the third shift in estimating the number of employees needed for each shift. The team assumed that the workload, percentage of stat tests, and distribution of test types would remain constant. It used a multiplier of 1.22 to have adequate staff for holidays, vacation, and illness. The team calculated an additional number of employees required for nonbench supporting activities such as quality control, preventive maintenance, ordering, inventory, and training, based on current usage.

The group used this approach to determine the number of technologists required on the third shift, then on the second shift, and finally on the first shift. The team estimated a time line for cross-coverage based on the laboratory's ongoing experience, and provided a sample rotational schedule. It calculated an annual employee turnover of 4.4%, based on our recent history.

From its report, the number, likely responsibilities, and thus background of employees required for the core laboratory were determined.

MANAGEMENT STRUCTURE (PART I)

While the staffing and space teams were at work, RISC began to discuss the difficult issue of management. The first important decision was to focus only on the core laboratory. While there was no a priori new organizational structure, we were aiming at a flexible, nimble unit that performed routine operations well but that was prepared to "shift gears" to take advantage of opportunities or minimize threats. We believed that this type of organization would be required to prosper in the future. Thus, we aimed at "flattening" the organizational structure by reducing the bureaucracy between top management and the bench worker. We thought we could best gauge the minimal levels needed after introducing, observing, and benchmarking new processes. We anticipated evolving the management structure from the processes themselves. This approach had been suggested by the consultants from Belcan Engineering as well as in discussions with faculty members from the school of industrial management.

RISC followed the familiar process of gathering all ideas through brainstorming to define those events required to develop a management structure in the core laboratory and then condensing the 16 items into 5 categories through an affinity process. The categories were (1) define the core laboratory, (2) identify the required staffing, (3) define the boundaries between the core laboratory and the rest of the laboratory, (4) list the functions of management in the core-laboratory, and (5) determine the relationship and integration of the core laboratory management with that of the entire laboratory. RISC also arranged these five categories by time requirements (Figure 5-4). We had defined the core laboratory, identified the staffing required, and were working on

We were aiming at a flexible, nimble unit that performed routine operations well but which was prepared to "shift gears" to take advantage of opportunities.

We aimed at "flattening" the organizational structure by reducing the bureaucracy between top management and the bench worker.

the core- and noncore-laboratory boundaries. Integration into the laboratory as a whole would be taken up later. We therefore focused on management functions in the core laboratory.

The specific items to be determined included the role of the supervisor in the core laboratory, the number of layers of management, the structure required to best serve the hospital and the medical center, the lines of authority, oversight of the work stations, and, perhaps most critical, the role of the faculty in the core laboratory.

The team concluded that both technical supervisor (bench supervisor) and manager positions would be needed. At the next meeting, RISC came to the consensus that a single manager should be responsible for overall operations. While RISC was occupied by reviewing, discussing, altering, and agreeing to the staffing and space team reports, the team recognized the need to bring this phase of planning to a close. We decided to hold two 1/2-day retreats to bring together staffing, space, and management structure and set a time line for construction of the core laboratory. Others who had played important roles in the reengineering process were also invited to the retreat.

RETREAT

RISC set the following objectives for the retreat: (1) develop an action plan and time line, (2) define boundaries for a transition team, (3) finalize the core laboratory management structure, (4) answer questions raised by the staffing and space team reports, (5) consider all the issues together to determine if other needs should be addressed. We asked all the laboratory sections and staff to communicate to us, either in writing or through e-mail, any lingering questions or concerns. These were gathered by the senior laboratory manager and presented as the first agenda item at the retreat. After the facilitator reviewed the state of planning for the core laboratory, we began to list and discuss those remaining issues and pieces of information necessary before developing a time line. Most of this effort centered on the time required to remodel physically the central laboratory, given the current space concept. We had already received budgetary approval and hospital support but now needed to determine from the hospital's physical plant section its estimate of remodeling time and costs. The space team had included one member from the physical plant section in its meetings so we knew the changes were possible and overall, modest. We were to receive an estimate of time at the second 1/2-day retreat to be held in 2 weeks. The group endorsed the space and staffing reports, including the need to move ahead with the specimen handling system.

After accepting the revised space and staffing reports, the retreat participants supported the need for an operations or "transition" team

Items to be determined included the role of the supervisor in the core laboratory, the number of layers of management, the structure required to best serve the hospital.

RISC came to a consensus that a single manager should be responsible for overall operations.

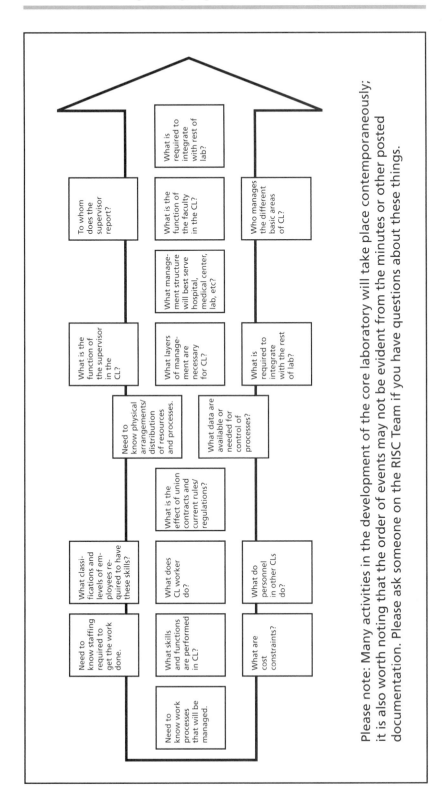

Figure 5-4.
Time line for the development of the management structure of the core laboratory (CL).

to be named to expedite the change from our current laboratory to a "core laboratory." The laboratory director, senior laboratory manager, director of quality assurance, and hospital space authority were directed to develop the transition team charge before the next 1/2-day retreat.

Management proposals that defined the roles of faculty members, managers, and technical supervisors were discussed. Based on the number of functions and clusters of work stations absorbed by the core laboratory, the group concluded that at least five managers would be needed. We also listed and discussed the pros and cons of whether a faculty member should be the director.

The group concluded that at least five managers would be needed.

Two weeks later, the members of the retreat regrouped for another 1/2-day meeting. At this session, the key characteristics of the person responsible for managing the core laboratory were discussed in detail. The senior laboratory manager was asked to prepare a draft of those characteristics, ie, a position description, for the next regularly scheduled RISC meeting. We reiterated the need for five core laboratory managers. The group concluded that it could not determine the number of technical supervisors required and that this would be best left to the managers, based on the number and nature of the work stations.

The process by which employees would be chosen for the core laboratory was delineated.

The process by which employees would be chosen for the core laboratory was delineated, ie, select employees based on job descriptions, qualifications, and laboratory needs and adhere to the state administrative code and contractual obligations. The specific skill groups and their positions were left to another team to be named.

The transition team was to be appointed by June 1, 1995. The charge to this team was approved (Table 5-1). Its first chore was to develop a detailed time line for implementation with the following target dates: the specimen handling system installed in 7 to 9 months, remodeling completed in 9 months, and opening of the core laboratory in 9 months. The timing for the specimen handling system was provided by the manufacturer with several months added by our staff for testing and reconstruction. The timing for remodeling was provided by the hospital's physical plant personnel with an increase of 50% added by the laboratory staff.

We were inextricably committed to this new adventure.

Finally, there was a consensus that this was a "go" and that we were inextricably committed to this new adventure.

MANAGEMENT STRUCTURE (PART II)

The position description of the core laboratory manager/director included administrative, educational, and research and development responsibilities. This person would report directly to the laboratory director and the senior laboratory manager. The description was presented to RISC at the first session after the retreat. Members were generally pleased by the document and were asked to submit comments or changes directly to its pri-

PROPOSED CHARGE TO THE TRANSITION TEAM — Table 5-1.

Implement approved stage 1 plan for the core laboratory to include:

Development and monitoring of detailed times, including:
- Space demolition and remodeling
- Installation of specimen handling system
- Staging of ongoing testing
- Integration of new analytic systems
- Establishment of training programs
- Development of position descriptions
- Modeling of work schedules

Establishment of new policies and procedures, including:
- Position descriptions
- Human resources policies
- Training
- Specimen handling
- Uniform quality management
- Enhanced computer support

Monitor and evaluate performance, including:
- Turnaround time for tests
- Percent of testing performed in core laboratory

Authorize and appoint consultants and teams to:
- Implement specific items of the plan
- Obtain more detailed information

Communicate plans and actions to laboratory colleagues, hospital administration, RISC, and laboratory administration—including responding to inquiries.

Transfer management responsibilities from the transition team to the permanent operations managers of the core laboratory.

---

mary author, the senior laboratory manager. The specifics of the core-laboratory management structure was to be determined by a transition team, appointed by the laboratory director. The director of data processing was asked to head the transition team and later to become acting director of the core laboratory during the transition. Other transition team members included the senior laboratory manager and supervisors from chemistry, hematology, microbiology, and special chemistry with staffing from data processing and quality assurance.

At the last meeting before summer 1995, RISC reviewed the action plan and developed a list of potential impediments to completion of phase 1 renovations. The three major obstacles were considered to be (1) union contracts, (2) State of Wisconsin administrative code, and (3) adequate computer support.

The transition team had already held one meeting and was prepared to move ahead to meet the laboratory's ambitious deadlines.

STAFF DISCUSSIONS BY DIRECTOR

The management staff of the laboratory was concerned about keeping the rest of the laboratory informed.

The management staff of the laboratory was concerned about keeping the rest of the laboratory informed about future plans for the core laboratory and beyond. Thus, the reports from the space and staffing teams were distributed to laboratory personnel about a week before the laboratory director initiated a series of six small group meetings to include all members of the laboratory. These took place during the late spring and early summer of 1995 to discuss the following seven topics:

- A listing of assays to be done in the core laboratory and the rationale for their inclusion

- Current plans for changing the physical space to accommodate the core laboratory

- Names of those on the transition team

- Management structure for the core laboratory, ie, a "chief" with five managers plus technical supervisors to "coach" the clusters of activities

- What assays and space are not included in the core laboratory

- Numbers of personnel expected to work in the core laboratory; the criteria for selection, and the mode of training, ie, by activity cluster

- We would review the rest of the laboratory assays, sections, space, and management structure while the core laboratory was being constructed

INITIATION OF PLANS FOR THE REST OF THE LABORATORY

During the summer of 1995, the laboratory advisory group discussed the management structure for the rest of the laboratory. First, we determined that we needed to complete the organizational plan by the time the core laboratory was to open, ie, March 1, 1996. Further, we believed that RISC was the appropriate group to discuss and formulate the structure. Each section was reviewed as to its current status and the effects it would experience because of the core laboratory. These sections fell into two large groupings, those significantly reduced by the core laboratory and those substantially unchanged by the core laboratory. Although those falling in the latter grouping each had different issues of workload and supervision, it was time for those in the other grouping to be reconstituted or terminated. While structural issues were important, they were judged to be less vital than the human issues of developing and determining roles for the current faculty and managers. We began to develop a plan whereby the faculty and managers, ultimately together, would discuss their roles, their relation to the sections, the laboratory, and to each other. The director of quality assurance agreed to lead a series of such discussions that would also consider the interrelationships of the other sections of the laboratory to the core laboratory and to each other.

While structural issues were important, they were judged to be less vital than the human issues.

TRANSITION TEAM

The transition team, named by the laboratory director in early June 1995, was given the formidable charge of fleshing out all the details required to make the core laboratory a reality. Key to accomplishing this mission was the change of reporting lines from the individual section managers to those who would exercise that role in the core laboratory. The transition team was given the authority to assume the role of the core-laboratory management in embryo until a permanent structure was determined.

The director of data processing was the chair of the transition team, so appointed because of his continued involvement in and contributions to the reengineering effort. The other members included seven senior medical technologists from each of the four services most affected by the core laboratory plus the senior laboratory manager, the technologist charged with process analysis, and a union representative. The course of events could not be anticipated, and the medical technologist who eventually became the administrator of the core laboratory was not included on the team. Because of necessity, the team had an amount of authority to which most of its members were unaccustomed, and there was a certain amount of apprehension about making decisions that would have a major impact on the future of the core laboratory and potentially the division of laboratory medicine as a whole.

Space/Ergonomics

The first technical challenge for the team was developing a third dimension for the floor plan of the core laboratory. Bench layouts needed to

The first technical challenge was developing a third dimension for the floor plan of the core laboratory.

be refined to indicate bench height, the location of kneeholes, the types of under-bench cabinets, the utilities that were required at the bench surface, and the above-bench shelving. This task required that the nature of the work to be performed at each work station be given at least a preliminary analysis. After this analysis, the team conducted an inventory of all existing cabinet and bench units in the laboratory or storage with the thought that these would be available for reallocation. This list allowed the team to draft a list of items to be purchased. Simultaneously, employees from the hospital's physical plant were determining their needs for construction materials. One technologist was assigned the overall responsibility for identifying and ordering needed materials.

The development of the third dimension of the core laboratory was strongly influenced by health concerns. To prevent repetitive motion injuries, fatigue, and muscle strains, the team reviewed ergonomic guidelines for laboratory construction and attempted to incorporate ergonomic improvements without undue cost or construction problems. We were also concerned about the noise level in the open area of the core laboratory with its increased personnel and large equipment. Two consultants, one from the university and one from industry, could not be certain that a noise problem would exist and recommended a wait-and-see attitude. We also started to evaluate the handling of waste materials, including trash. These efforts were significant but resulted in few changes because better alternatives could not be identified or were not commercially available.

Specimen Handling System

A specimen handling system was a key ingredient in the core-laboratory design.

The installation of a specimen handling system (see Figure 5-5) was a key ingredient in the core-laboratory design. We had decided on the use of such an overhead transport system early in the work of the space team, but getting a contract to install the system was a difficult and time-consuming process. The system had to be custom-made, and, because of budgetary constraints, there were few vendors interested in the project. Moreover, the University of Wisconsin Hospital and Clinics (UWHC) purchasing department was inexperienced in purchasing something that was part instrument and part building component. The result was a series of internal delays that slowed the bidding of the system. In the meantime, we obtained unofficial estimates of the cost from two potential suppliers, and several changes in the proposed system were made to reduce the cost. The bid was finally held in September 1995, but at the meeting to review the required specifications and bid ground rules, the putative "bidders" from industry were unable to meet the specifications and terms as described. The result was a series of changes and the receipt of only one viable bid, that being from Dorner Manufacturing

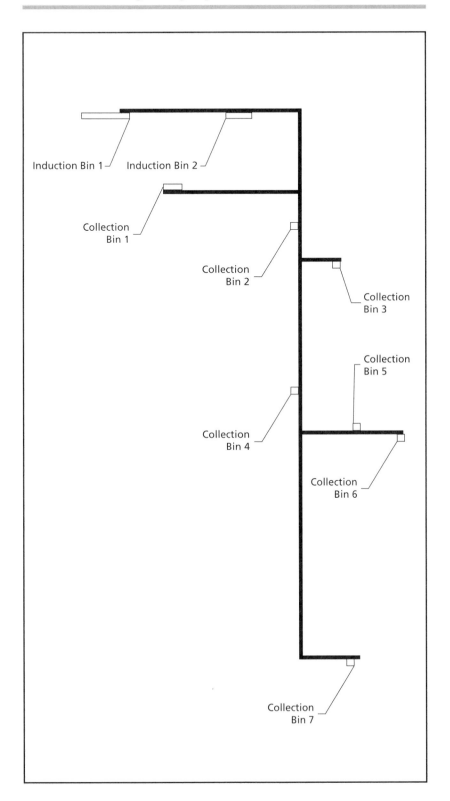

Figure 5-5.
Top view of the layout of the specimen handling system showing the positions of the two upstations and seven downstations. The system is ceiling mounted and is 64 feet long and 37 feet wide.

Company (Hartland, Wis). Because even this bid did not completely meet the hospital's stipulations, there was a 5-month-long negotiation process resulting in a contract award in May 1996. The specimen handling system was delivered about 9 months later in February 1997.

During the negotiations surrounding purchase of the specimen handling system, the laboratory staff expressed great concern about the capability of the system to perform the task of transporting specimen tubes successfully and safely. There were five major areas of doubt, as follows:

The laboratory staff expressed great concern about the capability of the system.

- Would the conveyor and sorting system break the specimen tubes?

- Would the movement of the tubes through the system damage the integrity of the patient samples?

- Would the system produce excessive noise?

- Would the system accurately and reliably read the barcodes on the tubes?

- Would the system be durable with few breakdowns?

We addressed these legitimate concerns as directly as possible. On three occasions the laboratory staff had induction bins, the input stations of the specimen handling system, brought to the clinical laboratory to test specimen integrity and tube breakage. The results of these tests indicated tubes would not be broken and that test results would not be altered by handling. The noise produced by the induction bins was not considered excessive. The other concerns could not be addressed until the unit was installed. For example, we had to make minor alterations to the pneumatic pushers to quiet the process of moving tubes to the down conveyors. The read-failure turned out to be 0.1%. Durability can be assessed only after more field experience.

Given the problems in acquiring the specimen handling system, we were not able to adhere to our initial time line. While the transition team was able to meet deadlines dependent only on the laboratory, it was unable to do so when the critical pathway involved external (hospital or supplier) performance. Thus, the goal of opening the core laboratory by March 1996 soon was pushed back to April 15. One of the team members was placed in charge of time line management, but so many things happened in the first few months to disrupt the rough time line that the overall project soon became a group of free-flowing subprojects. We continued to move forward on as many fronts as rapidly as possible, even though that movement was not as coordinated as we might have liked.

Construction

The execution of the construction plan was logistically difficult. The core laboratory was to be created in 7000 square feet of prime laboratory space, an area occupied by chemistry, special coagulation, specimen receiving, hematology, and send-outs. This area contained much of the laboratory's ongoing activities. We did not have access to other space to move these functions while the core laboratory was being constructed. Therefore, we built the new laboratory at the same time that laboratory work was being performed. This meant reoccurring episodes of service relocation as each area was redeveloped.

We built the new laboratory at the same time that laboratory work was being performed.

We named two contact people to interact with the craftsmen working on the project. One of these was the transition team member most involved with developing the detailed construction plans and the other, a nonteam member who eventually became the core-laboratory administrator. This move limited the duplicity of instructions given the craftsmen and was a success until the construction supervisor for the hospital's physical plant retired and was not replaced during the project. Therefore, 4 months into the project, each of the trades began working independently of each other.

Construction began in October 1995, approximately 3 months behind the initial schedule. In phase I, one side of the hematology laboratory was vacated and the area rebuilt for special coagulation. This phase went smoothly and met the revised schedule (see floor plan). When it was completed, the special coagulation operation was moved into place, and its previous space was renovated for specimen processing (phase II). This was the point at which the physical plant supervisor retired and our well-developed coordination plans became inoperative. For example, construction supplies did not arrive in a timely manner, preventing the area from being completed. Parts of this phase were finished a year after their scheduled completion date. Phase III, the construction of the center of the core laboratory, was launched in January 1996.

Phase III required vacating 3000 square feet in the center of the main laboratory and closing the specimen receiving window. All the benches and interior walls were removed—a dusty and noisy process but anticipated. Unforeseen was a 2-month delay caused by the need to place new drains into the floor with drain pipes buried 5 feet below ground level. The demolition of the work floor was followed by trenching and recementing. The remainder of construction proceeded at a more predictable pace.

Moving instruments into the core laboratory required personnel training and resolution of process and control issues. We had planned staff training to be done at specified times when we had maximal staff levels, ie, when few employees were on vacation and there were few medical

The construction delay prevented us from using the best opportunity for training.

technology students in the laboratory. The construction delay prevented us from using the best opportunity for training. Thus, little cross-training had been accomplished when construction finally permitted the workstations to be established in their permanent locations. In addition, the absence of the specimen handling system and a continuously changing work configuration severely hampered process redesign. The initial efforts to run the core laboratory was therefore adversely affected by the amount of "firefighting" that had to be done just to maintain routine operations. Because much of the construction and workstation movement occurred during the periods when students were present and during the summer vacation months only made a difficult situation worse.

Pressure by the hospital administration to withdraw what they now regarded as "excess" personnel as soon as vacancies occurred further retarded the efforts.

Pressure by the hospital administration to withdraw what they now regarded as "excess" personnel as soon as vacancies occurred further retarded the efforts to occupy the new space in a work-efficient manner. Despite this, our laboratory staff, although severely stressed, was able to maintain patient services without noticeable interruption.

Personnel/Management

The personnel situation was the most troubling of all the problems.

The personnel situation was the most troubling of all the problems that we had to address. We had negotiated a memorandum of understanding with the union to facilitate the transfer of personnel from their previous assignments to the core laboratory. The transition team established a work group to survey employees on their preferences and to decide who would be moved and who would remain in their current positions. We established the guideline that the burden of weekend coverage should be distributed as uniformly as possible across the laboratory. The personnel work group distributed its questionnaire at a series of laboratory information sessions conducted by laboratory management at the end of September 1995. All employees were asked to indicate whether they would be willing to work in the core laboratory and if so, under what conditions. The committee tabulated the results, which were then to define personnel assignments during the next 6 months. The immediate assignment of personnel, however, was inhibited by two other factors.

While the organizational structure of the core laboratory had been outlined, the process for filling these positions had not been completed, mainly because it was unclear how best to comply with the State of Wisconsin administrative code. Thus, there had been no permanent appointments to the core-laboratory management. In mid–August 1995, the chair of the transition team was asked to serve as the acting director of the core laboratory. This was to be a 1-year appointment until a permanent structure had been developed. At that time, the transition team assumed responsibility for decisions on testing in the core laboratory.

The transition team assumed responsibility for decisions on testing in the core laboratory.

In September 1995, the laboratory director resigned at the request of the new chair of pathology, and both the department of pathology and laboratory medicine and the clinical laboratory were restructured. Hospital administration agreed in principle to reorganize the entire laboratory into four administrative areas, with medical technologists rather than faculty members serving as the area administrators. At this time, University Hospital and Clinics was moving toward becoming a public authority and no longer being a part of the University of Wisconsin—Madison. While agreeing to the organizational change in principle, the UWHC administration was undecided on how these positions were to be filled, thus preventing a permanent core-laboratory management from being appointed for more than a year and making it difficult to appoint even a temporary management structure. In the meantime, the transition team continued to act as the core-laboratory management, working in parallel with the managements of the various laboratory sections that were still in place.

The second factor influencing the personnel division among the laboratory areas and sections was the lack of a staffing model for the core laboratory or any of the rest of the laboratory sections that would be greatly affected by the establishment of the core laboratory. To attempt to get a handle on how the resources of the laboratory would have to be divided in this new management model, we appointed an organizational team for each of the four management areas. Of all these teams, the core-laboratory team was the most successful because its mission was the easiest to grasp. Under the leadership of a member of the transition team who was a leading candidate to become the administrator of the core laboratory, the team refined the work of previous personnel teams and incorporated much more detail into its staffing model. Based on this model, we finally were able to consider the redeployment of the laboratory staff.

By December 1995, we had arrived at a critical point in our effort to create the core laboratory. While construction was proceeding in the second of the five phases, the fact that neither area administrators, supervisors, nor staff had yet been assigned to any of the tasks created an atmosphere of uncertainty and pessimism that threatened the whole project. We therefore asked the transition team to hold an intense working session that lasted nearly a week. In addition to the regular members, several other senior members of the laboratory technical staff were invited to discuss how to distribute the personnel and how positions would be structured. Using standard total quality management (TQM) techniques, all the positions in the laboratory that could be affected by the creation of the core laboratory were discussed one at a time. Differing ideas about the methods of the changes were debated, and a

In September 1995, the laboratory director resigned at the request of the new chair of pathology and both the department of pathology and laboratory medicine and the clinical laboratory were restructured.

By December 1995, we had arrived at a critical point in our effort to create the core laboratory.

All the positions in the laboratory that could be affected by the creation of the core laboratory were discussed.

general understanding of what had to be done was gained by everyone involved, even though the interpretation of how the details would be addressed still differed.

In January 1996, the laboratory and hospital administrations named acting administrators for the four areas of the laboratory. The senior laboratory manager was asked to oversee administrative services, while the other three areas were assigned to the chief technologists from chemistry (core laboratory), hematology (special services), and microbiology (emerging technology). Shortly after the appointment of the new leadership, the transition team was dissolved because its membership and mission overlapped that of the new area administrators. The laboratory began the formal transition to the new administrative structure, which coincided with the empowerment of the hospital as a public authority at the end of June 1996.

The laboratory began the formal transition to the new administrative structure, which coincided with the empowerment of the hospital as a public authority at the end of June 1996.

Other Issues

The transition team had planned to address systematically all the processes within the core laboratory through the formation of work groups. Because of the factors given above, this was not possible and process improvement was left for core-laboratory management to address as part of ongoing operations.

Like process improvement, cross-training was a task we had delegated to the transition team. This too could not be completed in the scheduled time and it was left to core-laboratory management to do that training.

The development of computer software specifically aimed at core-laboratory issues was also delayed but eventually completed in early 1997.

We also needed to review our use of the telephone and gave a work group extensive latitude in proposing solutions. In the end, however, the cost of a versatile telephone system was not feasible, and most elements of the previous phone system were retained. The phone center continued to receive all business calls during the day shift, and its incoming number was transferred to the core laboratory during off-shifts. Personal calls were directed to two phones established for that purpose on opposite sides of the laboratory.

The transition team made dramatic progress in the completion of the core laboratory.

The transition team had only begun to address the different cultures of the five laboratory areas that formed the core laboratory. For example, integrating employee break areas from a separate one for each section to "merged" sites took time and consideration.

In retrospect, the transition team made dramatic progress in the completion of the core laboratory despite the obstacles it faced. Considering both the administrative and construction turmoil, the plan that the RISC gave it was faithfully followed. Delays came from the outside and not from the failure of the team to maintain good project management. The delays, however, caused many problems for the team, because they removed the level of urgency needed to get the task completed. In place of urgency came frustration caused by slow to no progress and the degree of disruption. Many personnel lost confidence in the project and were disturbed by the uncertainty of not knowing their future roles in the laboratory and not even the laboratory's future role in the hospital. This led to political jostling and insecurity among some members of the team. Although the transition team handed the completion of the project to others in January 1996, the plan it created for the implementation remained to a large degree intact and guided the completion of the core laboratory.

Delays came from the outside and not from the failure of the team.

Lessons Learned

INTRODUCTION

Total quality management (TQM) is effective but not easily accomplished. There is no simple TQM formula that ensures success. There are, however, guiding principles, including Deming's 14 points,[1] which enhance the likelihood of obtaining positive results.

The application of the scientific method to management is the heart and soul of TQM; plan, do, check, act or standardize, and then cycle again. Benchmarking is the central nervous system, the brain, of TQM. If you cannot measure a process, you will not know if you have improved it. The tools provide a systematic disciplined approach to improving a process, and training in these tools allows team members with varying backgrounds to participate.

Application of the scientific method to management is the heart and soul of TQM.

If you cannot measure a process, you will not know if you have improved it.

At the inception of a TQM program, employees almost always complain about the time needed to initiate and implement TQM; however, in our experience the time is well spent. Problems are identified and solved rather than being allowed to fester. It takes time to solve most problems, but in the long run, it takes less time than the usual top-down approaches that often end in only temporary fixes rather than true solutions. TQM is often implemented to gain an advantage in a marketplace. There are, however, no guarantees of success in any business endeavor. The world is competitive and one's rivals may have superior resources and also may be using TQM.

There are no guarantees of success in any business endeavor.

Finally, gaining and retaining the support of upper management is critical to the fulfillment of any program. While TQM can be started by pockets of individuals, its results cannot be fully realized unless upper management at least accepts its practice and allows the program to progress and its gains to be sustained.

PROCESS AND MANAGEMENT

We learned what other TQM groups have learned, ie, defining and understanding the organizational vision and mission is critical to decision making at all levels, ie, how well does this choice fit in with our vision/mission. We found that at times the vision and mission were understood without being put into words. Nevertheless, it would be desirable to have such documents at the beginning of a TQM adventure, but it is not absolutely necessary. What is necessary, however, is that the members of the organization think about and support the vision/mission.

We concur with others that by adhering to a plan, do, check, and act methodology, groups or teams almost always accomplish their goals. The end result may be greater than, and often different from, the outcome originally conceived. The program and the organization will gain by team training and approaching problems in a disciplined TQM process. Most of the members of a successful team will become advocates and teachers for other teams, geometrically increasing the influence of the program. The greatest difficulties for project teams are in defining a doable mission with appropriate benchmarks. The manufacturing sector produces "widgets," which are easily counted; however, service industries, such as in health care, have difficulty in defining their "widget" equivalents and then enumerating them. Clinical laboratories have the advantage of large quantities of data, much of which might be used to benchmark aspects of laboratory performance. In our situation, the difficulty was not the absence of data but the selection of which data were the most relevant to our projects. We would suggest scheduling the time needed to define a doable mission with available benchmarks.

The greatest difficulties for project teams are in defining a doable mission with appropriate benchmarks.

We found it advantageous to follow guidelines and house rules in our team meetings. Using an established process provided teams with a "fall back" position when they might otherwise be floundering. In addition, we always included an action plan with a time line that served as a reassuring "homebase" when the team seemed to be veering on an uncertain course. Rules of behavior provided teams with methods by which they could deal with nonproductive conduct. Of course, we learned rapidly which personnel were most likely to contribute positively to a team effort. As more employees were trained in TQM tools and techniques, we were more confident in placing more difficult members on a team with TQM-experienced people. Nevertheless, some staff members were never asked to join a team and some were asked to serve on many teams.

We always included an action plan with a time-line.

We also learned that management should not ignore an opportunity to do the obvious. For example, if a project team identifies an easily correctable problem as it collects data, management should be informed and allowed to make the correction as soon as possible. This is often called a "nugget" in the TQM literature, and we think it is sometimes ignored. TQM never calls for ignoring the obvious and forgoing the use of common sense.

TQM never calls for ignoring the obvious and forgoing the use of common sense.

It was helpful and perhaps essential for us to have an overall template such as the GOAL/QPC 10-step program to follow. When we were uncertain about how to proceed and needed to put our efforts into some context, it was reassuring to know that we were "on target," even if occasionally askew. Later, the Hammer and Champy reengineering concept provided us with a popular and accepted program that allowed us to gain support for making more dramatic and necessary changes.

It should be apparent that we see reengineering as an extension of TQM and that we have used TQM improvement methodology, the team process, and the TQM problem-solving and planning tools to accomplish reengineering. We believe that TQM is a prerequisite to reengineering and essential for a successful outcome under the complex and demanding conditions of a laboratory operation such as ours. This does not imply that reengineering is easy with TQM; however, without a background in TQM and training in project methodology and team skills, reengineering is much more difficult.

We see reengineering as an extension of TQM.

Our clinical laboratories gathered enormous quantities of data for various reasons. Although this was far more than most other health care and perhaps service sector units, we often found that the data were not exactly suitable for our project goals, nor were they complete enough. We sometimes had to collect more data or interpolate from existing information. Some things were difficult to quantify and we made best judgments in these areas rather than be prevented from proceeding at all. As projects developed, we recognized more appropriate measurements and improved the benchmarks.

It is helpful to have access to the efforts of others both in and out of health care because they might provide external benchmarks or ideas. For example, we learned about GOAL/QC initially through a Madison-based quality group, the Madison Area Quality Improvement Network. The local public television station sponsored management programs including several on reengineering. Cost and productivity data were available from the University Hospital Consortium and the College of American Pathologists (CAP).

In writing this book, we were grateful that we had placed so much emphasis on documenting our efforts. Teams maintained good minutes and notes. Drafts and final versions were easily identified. Dates were included with all documents. We could monitor progress with the use of action time lines. As new teams were initiated, they were greatly aided by reviewing earlier team documents.

We placed emphasis on documenting our efforts.

We learned that resources of time, space, people, and sometimes money were required. Thus, it was imperative that these resources be budgeted. In our case, this meant suggesting, supporting, and defending allocations in the hospital budget. In many organizations, budget preparation may be a fairly routine process from year-to-year. We suggest awareness of this process because if resources are not allocated or

A budget often dictate priorities rather than priorities dictating a budget.

reduced, the program will suffer. For better or worse, a budget often dictates priorities rather than priorities dictating a budget.

Finally, we cannot overemphasize the responsibility of management to communicate with all employees. With rare exception, communication should be open. Because we are both a public and a service organization, we did our best to share information with our employees. Thus, while we made progress over a 7-year period, the laboratory culture had not completely changed, and the hospital culture had not changed at all, to allow for trust in management and in each other.

HUMAN RESOURCES

Once employees are convinced that management is "serious" about TQM, most will contribute positively to the effort. Of course, most people would prefer to be on a team rather than stuck on the sidelines; however, we asked for more than compliance. TQM seeks contributions to the planning of work as well as doing work. We believe that this inclusion increases understanding of work processes, better decision making, and more effective work. The staff in the clinical laboratory responded positively to our efforts and contributed to its planning and implementation efforts, sometimes in the midst of difficult circumstances.

Inclusion increases understanding of work processes, better decision making, and more effective work.

We, as management, tried to change the culture to allow individual efforts toward a common goal to flourish. The importance of an organization's culture cannot be overemphasized in the success of TQM or any other management program. We also tried to convey that this was a shared adventure and that we were mutually committed to the program and to each other. We learned that analytical skills were not a substitute for human skills, ie, the sensitivity to the needs of others and the ability to appeal to those qualities that would motivate staff. Money is only one of many motivators and one that we found almost impossible to use in a large statewide organization where rules and budgets virtually precluded using dollars as a reward. We would have welcomed the opportunity to tie performance within TQM to rewards. We did establish a recognition program where contributors received a plaque made by volunteers within the laboratory.

OTHER RESOURCES

We have touched on other resources needed for a TQM program. The most important of these is time and thus patience. TQM programs are usually slow to take hold because of employee suspicion and inexperience. The organization will need to invest in time and leadership, perhaps hiring or training a facilitator and renting or purchasing flip-charts, writing utensils, and Post-it® Notes (3M, St Paul, Minn). Computers and software are also great, perhaps indispensable, aids.

We usually underestimated the time required for completion of the early projects. However, the time invested was compensated for by the number of creative solutions leading to a more effective, competitive organization. Many of these solutions led to increased productivity at little or no extra cost.

We had some experience with external consultants. The organization was never in a position to hire one of them to guide any major component of our program. We suspect that consultants can be of great help if they are knowledgeable and have the confidence of upper management. However, even with consultants, the success or failure of a program will lie with the commitment and resourcefulness of those within the organization and not those who make suggestions from the outside.

BEFORE EMBARKING ON A TQM/REENGINEERING ADVENTURE

We wrote this book in large part to be of some help to those who might be considering the use of TQM and/or reengineering. We cannot quantify the likelihood of success, but we can provide some insights into some issues related to success or failure. We have broken these into organizational and personal components.

Organizational

The people or persons to whom you report should be supportive or at least neutral. It is most helpful if your unit's efforts are only one part of a larger, sincere organizational program.

Your unit will need considerable authority and flexibility, particularly if there is no overall TQM program. Because TQM involves altering the culture, your unit will need to be able to do this through control of finances and budget as well as of the time, duties, promotion, hiring, and firing of personnel. The layer of management above your unit will need to provide some protection from external politics and pressures.

Your unit will need considerable authority and flexibility, particularly if there is no overall TQM program.

The organization may not be prepared for TQM if its management culture is heavily "top-down," dictatorial, or even abusive. If your unit cannot specify job descriptions, it will be difficult to alter the priorities and the culture. If the organizational budget does not include resources, it will be difficult to convince staff of the sincerity of the TQM effort.

If the organization's vision and mission are ambiguous, it may be an opportunity for change but more likely it may signal a confused, unstable business. If communication within the organization is lacking or, even worse, filled with miscommunication, it will be difficult to teach the new programs and gain the confidence of the staff. Finally, if upper

It is important to have some knowledge of the history and current culture of the organization.

management is threatened by the success of others and/or is obsessed with control, TQM will be viewed with suspicion. We think that it is important to have some knowledge of the history and current culture of the organization as well as a clear understanding of its vision, mission, and current goals.

Personal

TQM requires faith that things can get better, continually.

TQM/reengineering is probably not for everyone. Even before examining an organization's readiness, one should examine his or her own traits. TQM requires faith that things can get better, continually. It embraces the scientific method and reliance on data for decision making. Its tenets teach that others, at all levels, can be trained in TQM tools and techniques, that staff can work together toward common goals. TQM insists upon planning before implementation. Management must have the patience to look toward the "long haul," training its staff, allowing it to gain experience, making some mistakes. TQM teaches that by improving processes, one will improve work and that those closest to the process can contribute to improving it. It is hard work and not a trendy joy ride. Its rewards derive from unit improvements with contributions from almost all employees. It is more likely to develop smarter more committed staff and thus a smarter, organization, a learning organization. The structure of TQM is often depicted as an inverted triangle with the CEO at the bottom of the triangle rather than at the top as in the more traditional renditions of organizational structures. Each person must determine his or her own comfort level with this managerial role.

It is hard work and not a trendy joy ride.

REFERENCE

1. Deming WE. *Out of the Crisis.* Cambridge, Mass: Massachusetts Institute of Technology, Center for Advanced Study; 1987.

Appendix

Center for Health Sciences

Date: November 16, 1994
To: Laboratory Managers
From: Clinical Laboratory Directors

Health Care Reform—Our Role as the Division of Laboratory Medicine

Health care as we know it in this country is undergoing profound changes. All the forces that can be mustered from government, industry, market competition, and the like are converging to cause this upheaval. Hospitals everywhere are experiencing significant economic challenges; academic institutions such as ours face difficult strategic decisions. In this climate, all health care elements including clinical laboratories must critically reexamine their function and ensure that the form they take logically and cost-effectively follows that function.

Our purpose as the clinical laboratories is to provide a resource to the health care providers of this hospital so they can more adequately diagnose, manage, treat, and monitor their patients' conditions. Although the means of providing these services undergo constant revision and refinement, that basic tenet will not change. We cannot fulfill our purpose, however, if physicians do not bring their patients to this hospital or—what is more likely to be the problem in today's managed care environment—patients do not come because their managed care providers do not contract with our hospital for economic reasons. Hence, containing the costs of laboratory work is increasingly important. These realities have caused us to consider our options. Over the past 20 months, discussions have been held, investigative projects have gone forward, various reengineering teams on which some of you served performed valuable work, consultants were brought in, and reports were written. We are determined to be proactive in these endeavors rather than passive or, even worse, reactive. The goal is to restructure the laboratories to improve our efficiency so that we can maintain our respected service, continue to advance our practice of clinical laboratory science, and provide meaningful employment, all while containing our costs. We are convinced these objectives are achievable by reorganizing the laboratory based more on technology than on laboratory specialty, increasing our use of automation wherever possible, and forming a core laboratory where much of the higher volume, automated testing can be consolidated.

Following this cover letter is a report from a team charged with providing a financial analysis of a proposed "core laboratory." The specific suggestions in this document form a model of this approach and require further careful consideration before we implement any or all of the suggestions. We need your advice and involvement.

Hospital administration has agreed in principle with the general idea of forming a core laboratory. Money already has been set aside in this fiscal year's budget for possible renovation expenses. The core chemistry laboratory instrument bid process now underway also fits the reorganization plan we might implement. While it is true that some of our cost containment will be realized through staff reductions, hospital administration does not currently have plans for layoffs in the laboratory. Laboratory administration is committed to avoiding layoffs, reinvesting positions back into the laboratory whenever strategically necessary or back into the hospital in some suitable function, and giving up positions through attrition.

The outcome of health care reform is still uncertain. What is certain is that the status quo is no longer an option. We, as the professionals who manage and work in the clinical laboratories, have work to do. Fortunately, we also have the skills, talents, and other resources to accomplish our task.